TRAINING FOR OBSTACLE COURSE RACING

TRAIN LIKE A PRO

Series Editor: Will Peveler

Rowman & Littlefield's Train Like a Pro series provides nonprofessional athletes, coaches, and trainers with training guides based on scientifically backed information that is both easy to follow and readily implemented. Each book covers the equipment, basic training physiology, specific training techniques, and tips for building a training plan for a specific sport, as well as competition, nutrition, and special considerations. These books are especially beneficial for athletes who have to train while working full-time jobs, as they provide recommendations for how training can be built around a busy schedule.

Strength and Conditioning for Mixed Martial Arts: A Practical Guide for the Busy Athlete by Will Peveler (2021)

Training for Mountain Biking: A Practical Guide for the Busy Athlete by Will Peveler (2021)

Training for Obstacle Course Racing: A Practical Guide for the Busy Athlete by Will Peveler (2021)

TRAINING FOR OBSTACLE COURSE RACING

A Practical Guide for the Busy Athlete

Will Peveler

ROWMAN & LITTLEFIELD
Lanham • Boulder • New York • London

Published by Rowman & Littlefield
An imprint of The Rowman & Littlefield Publishing Group, Inc.
4501 Forbes Boulevard, Suite 200, Lanham, Maryland 20706
www.rowman.com

6 Tinworth Street, London, SE11 5AL, United Kingdom

British Library Cataloguing in Publication Information Available

Library of Congress Cataloging-in-Publication Data

Name: Peveler, Will, author.
Title: Training for obstacle course racing : a practical guide for the busy athlete / Will
    Peveler.
Description: Lanham, Maryland : Rowman & Littlefield, 2021. | Series: Train like a
    pro | Includes index. | Summary: "A training guide for the nonprofessional obstacle
    course racer, this book provides elite-level information that is easy to follow and
    readily implemented into a busy life schedule. It covers topics such as equipment
    selection, techniques for conquering specific obstacles, developing a training plan,
    proper nutrition, and more"—Provided by publisher.
Identifiers: LCCN 2020052939 (print) | LCCN 2020052940 (ebook) | ISBN
    9781538139585 (cloth) | ISBN 9781538139592 (ebook)
Subjects: LCSH: Obstacle racing—Training.
Classification: LCC GV1067 .P48 2021 (print) | LCC GV1067 (ebook) | DDC
    796.42/6—dc23
LC record available at https://lccn.loc.gov/2020052939
LC ebook record available at https://lccn.loc.gov/2020052940

CONTENTS

ACKNOWLEDGMENTS

I would like to thank my wife, Renee, and our four sons, Grayson, Garrett, Will, and LJ, for supporting me throughout the process of writing this book as well as the other books in the series. My wife was coerced into being in some of the photos as well as taking some of the photos for the book. My son Grayson was also hijacked to take some of the photos as well. Without the support of my family, I would not be able to do much of what I do.

Last but not least, I would like to thank my editors, Christen Karniski and Erinn Slanina, for working with me during this process, putting up with all my questions, and making me sound somewhat intelligent.

INTRODUCTION

The goal of the Train Like a Pro series is to provide elite-level training information that is easily understandable and implemented. Each book in the series will provide you with the following information on the sport: required equipment, a basic understanding of how the body responds and adapts to training, basic training principles, how to develop a training plan, exercise techniques, and basic sport nutrition for performance. Most professional athletes are paid to both train and compete, and therefore their lives are built around those work requirements. This series is written for nonprofessional athletes. The majority of individuals reading these books have jobs, families, and other responsibilities that prevent them from working their life around training and competition. Instead, they must find a way to work their training and competition into life. It is important to find a balance that allows you to work, have quality family time, and improve your performance.

The goal of *Training for Obstacle Course Racing* is to provide you with all the basic information to allow you to be successful in the sport of obstacle course racing (OCR). I wrote this book with beginners in mind. It provides information on equipment, training, nutrition, and competition—in short, all the basic information I wish I would have had prior to participating in my first obstacle course race. Whether you are a complete beginner or an experienced athlete, you will gain a lot of useful knowledge from this book.

WHY BECOME INVOLVED IN OCR?

Many people become involved in obstacle course racing because of the physical and mental challenges the sport provides. It allows you to push your perceived limits to discover what you are truly made of and what you can accomplish. Obstacle course racing first developed using the concept of military training. It allows civilians to push their mind and body to determine if they are up for the challenge. For many, just completing an obstacle course race is reward enough. For others, the primary drive is competition.

One of the unique aspects of obstacle course racing is that it is an individual sport. This allows athletes of varying ages and fitness levels to become involved. You can train and race at your own pace and on your own schedule (although it is always fun to train and race with friends!). Some events, however, encourage teams and teamwork. In some races, obstacles are made so that they are impossible to traverse on your own and will require teamwork.

Another unique factor of obstacle course racing is the nature of the obstacles themselves. Each obstacle will challenge a unique set of skills and attributes. The overall competition requires aerobic fitness, but anaerobic fitness, muscular strength, endurance, and power are also used throughout the course. These courses will also challenge your balance, skill sets, and fortitude. How to train for and conquer the most commonly seen obstacles will be covered in this book.

Health

Improved health is a great motivator for obstacle course racers. Many athletes become involved in OCR during their pursuit of a healthier lifestyle. Individuals who are physically active are four times less likely to develop cardiovascular disease than those who do not participate in regular physical exercise. This fact is so strongly supported by available research that the American College of Sports Medicine recently implemented the Exercise is Medicine initiative, which is officially supported by the U.S. surgeon general.

Obstacle course racing provides a challenging but attainable goal for those who wish to get in shape for health or personal reasons. To maximize the health benefits of exercise, 30 minutes of physical activity per day is recommended for most days of the week. During training you will exceed those minimum recommendations and be well on your way to the development of a lifelong healthy lifestyle.

While physical activity has a strong positive impact on your health, you must first ensure that you are healthy enough to begin an exercise program with no restrictions. Exercise takes your body out of homeostasis (the maintenance of balance within the human body: body temperature, blood glucose levels, etc.) and therefore increases the risk of a cardiovascular incident in those with undiagnosed or unknown heart conditions. You should seek a physician's clearance prior to beginning an exercise program in order to confirm that you are healthy enough to train. This is especially true for sedentary individuals, older individuals, those who have not had a recent physical, and those with signs of or risk factors for the development of cardiovascular disease.

Racing

Many individuals become involved in obstacle course racing for the competitive aspect. They enjoy pushing their body, mind, and resolve to the limits. While you will be racing against other individuals, the real race is with yourself, to determine if you are better today than you were yesterday. Racing provides an opportunity to push yourself harder than you would in training, and many people thrive on that feeling. However, not all obstacle course races are timed for competition. Many just focus on the completion of the course.

HOW TO GET INVOLVED

Big Race Brands

The market for OCR has grown exponentially over the last 10 years and is now more mainstream, making it easy to find information on upcoming races. One of the best ways is to look up the main OCR brands and examine the race schedule for the year. At the time of writing this book the top race brands are Spartan, Tough Mudder, and Rugged Maniac. All three of these organizations provide well-supported races with amazing challenges. The pricing for these races is considered expensive, but you must take into account the cost of the obstacles, maintenance of the equipment, setup of each race, venue fees, and liability insurance.

You can also find regional races that are run by local organizations. Many times, these races may not have the same level of obstacles as the larger races, but they are typically less expensive and just as much fun. Do not discount a race just because it is not from one of the larger organizations.

Local OCR Club

A great place to find information on OCR would be a local OCR club. There will be many experienced racers who would be more than willing to help you get started. If there are multiple clubs in your area, try a few out to see which is the best fit for you and your OCR goals. You can find information about your local OCR club through social media or through your local running store. If your area does not have an OCR club, try a local running club as they most likely will have members who are involved in OCR racing, and consider starting your own OCR club.

GEAR FOR OBSTACLE COURSE RACING

There is not a lot of required gear to participate in OCR. However, you do need some specialized gear for both training and racing. Some of the training gear can be purchased or built, or you can join a gym that has the necessary equipment. This book will cover the equipment you will need for competing in and training for obstacle course racing.

TRAINING AND NUTRITION

To successfully participate in OCR, it is vital that you develop and maintain a sound training and nutrition plan. It is important to develop a plan that incorporates different volumes and intensities along with appropriate recovery time in order to optimize performance while preventing overtraining. As OCR requires aerobic capacity, anaerobic capacity, muscular endurance, muscular strength, muscular power, and flexibility, it is important to incorporate all these components into your training program. Most individuals reading this book will have jobs, families, and other responsibilities, and these factors must be taken into consideration when developing a training program. This book will help you develop a basic training plan that will allow you to improve performance without overtraining.

While most OCR racers spend a lot of time developing their training plan, they commonly ignore their nutrition plan. To optimize training, you must not only eat specific types of food but also consider the amount of food and the timing of meals. Your nutritional plan is just as important as your training plan.

1

EQUIPMENT

Obstacle course racing requires very little equipment compared to other sports. However, it is important to have a strong understanding of what is required so that you can better choose the appropriate equipment. This chapter is designed to provide the information needed when purchasing gear for obstacle course racing.

RUNNING SHOES

Before talking about proper shoes, it is important to discuss running and ground reaction forces. It is critical that you gain an understanding of these forces in order to truly understand the importance of choosing appropriate running shoes. Ground reaction forces occur when the foot makes contact with the ground while running. The ground reaction force is equal and opposite in direction to the force applied to the ground (Newton's third law of action–reaction) and is based on the individual's mass, the acceleration of gravity, and running speed. The ground reaction forces in running are typically two to three times the individual's body weight, but can reach up to five times the body weight at high speeds. While this force is necessary to propel the body forward, it also must be absorbed up the kinetic chain every time the foot strikes the ground. Repetitive ground reaction forces and the resultant biomechanical response as force is applied up the kinetic chain is the main reason for injuries due to running. While the primary method for absorbing the ground reaction forces is biomechanical in nature, proper running shoes can also assist in absorbing impact.

While the ground reaction forces of each ground contact may not seem like much, consider how many times each foot strikes the ground during a run. The average runner will run at about 150 steps per minute, and an elite runner may run at about 180 steps per minute. For a one-hour run, that would result in 9,000 (60 min × 150 steps) to 10,800 (60 min × 180 steps) steps. These repetitive forces lead to a large amount of stress placed on the bones and joints of the body. This is why understanding running biomechanics and shoe choice becomes extremely important.

The most vital piece of equipment that you will purchase for obstacle course racing is your running shoes. Running in improper shoes can not only be uncomfortable but lead to overuse injuries that can negatively impact training. Due to my background, I have had many athletes come to me with questions regarding training. One common question I get from beginning runners deals with leg pain—mainly lower leg pain (ankle, shin, and knee). After a short conversation, we usually discover two common factors. The first concerns the individual increasing intensity or duration too quickly, which is easily modified through altering their training schedule (and usually means developing one). The second concern typically deals with the fact that they are running in improper shoes. Some common issues with the shoes are:

- Running in shoes that are not designed for running, such as court shoes. Court shoes, such as basketball shoes, are designed to make quick lateral movements on a court surface, whereas running shoes are designed primarily for forward movement. Due to this, court shoes make a poor choice for running shoes.
- Training in running shoes that are old and well past their usefulness. The old running shoes that you have been mowing the yard in for the last three years are not a good choice for training.
- Running in new shoes that are not designed for that person's particular biomechanics. This can lead to overuse injuries.
- Shoes that do not fit correctly.

Choosing the Correct Shoes

When purchasing new shoes, it is important to choose a pair that best fits your needs, your budget, and most importantly your individual anthropometrics and biomechanics. There are two key factors when choosing appropriate running shoes. The first deals with your body mass, and the second deals with the manner in which you run. The first of these two considerations is the easiest to address. As your weight increases, the need for a more cushioned shoe will also increase. The second consideration is a little more complicated.

The interaction of the foot and the ground is extremely important in regard to running. There are two basic phases of the lower extremities during running. The first phase of running is the stance phase, which contains three distinct subphases. The first subphase begins when the heel strikes the ground in a slightly supinated position. The next subphase of the stance phase, midstance, occurs as the midfoot moves forward to contact the ground; as this movement occurs the foot will move into pronation. Toe off, the last subphase, occurs as the foot leaves the ground. When the foot leaves the ground, there will be a brief period of time where neither foot is on the ground. This is referred to as the flight phase. The phases listed above are considered "normal"; however, there are variations. Some runners will have less of a heel strike, while others will have more. At this point, we will concentrate more on pronation (the foot rolling toward the midline of your body) and supination (the foot rolling away from the midline of your body). While there are many variations, there are three basic categories that runners fall into: in line, overpronation, or supination.

In-line or neutral runners follow the basic outline of the stance phase listed above with little variation. They typically have a normal arch and do not excessively pronate. Due to this, a neutral-cushion shoe is recommended for these runners. A neutral-cushion shoe will provide cushioning and is built on a semicurved sole.

Everyone pronates when walking and running. This action is used to help absorb some of the ground reaction forces. However, overpronation, the foot rolling toward the midline excessively, may be an issue for some runners, and in many cases should be addressed. When the foot overpronates, it alters running kinematics and can lead to overuse injuries in runners. A motion-control shoe that provides medial support and is built on a straight sole is designed for this situation. Those who slightly overpronate, however, may be better served in a stability shoe that provides slight medial support. The typical cause of overpronation is lack of a normal arch. However, lack of flexibility and muscular imbalances or muscle weakness can also lead to overpronation. It is important to understand the cause in order to best address the problem. While a motion-control shoe will assist those who overpronate due to lack of a normal arch, it may not help if the overpronation is caused due to lack of flexibility, muscular weakness, or muscular imbalances. Also keep in mind that elite-level runners overpronate in order to better absorb the high ground reaction forces due to the high turnover rate they produce while running.

Individuals who supinate (run on the outside of the foot) will typically have a high arch, which forces the foot to the outside as they run. A cushioned shoe built on a curved sole is ideal for supinators. The curved sole and lack of medial support encourages the foot to pronate during the stance phase.

Barefoot or minimalist running has become popular in recent history. Barefoot or, more correctly termed, minimalist shoes are designed to have very little protection between the sole of your foot and the ground in order to promote "natural" running. The idea behind the theory is that the human foot was naturally designed to absorb ground reaction forces by running mid- to front foot and that wearing a minimalist shoe will encourage this type of running. A minimalist shoe will provide greater proprioceptive feedback in order to adjust to the terrain and will allow the foot more freedom of movement through the stance phase. A traditional running shoe is designed to protect against impact when the heel strikes the ground. However, because the heel is built up in the shoe, it also encourages the heel to strike the ground first. A traditional shoe also has less freedom of movement than a minimalist shoe during the stance phase and prevents meaningful proprioceptive feedback from ground contact. The benefit to a traditional shoe from this point of view is that the runner worries less about injury due to the terrain and can concentrate more on running the race. These are the fundamental differences between traditional running shoes and minimalist running shoes. As obstacle course racing is conducted on trails, I strongly recommend not running in minimalist shoes as they do not provide adequate foot protection on the run.

For obstacle course racing, you must also consider the sole of the shoe. Obstacle course racing requires running through mud and water where maximal traction is needed. All the climbing obstacles in a race course will require good traction from your feet as well as your hands. Therefore, choose good trail shoes that have a knobby sole tread that provides traction while not easily becoming clogged with mud. This makes road-running shoes impractical during obstacle course racing. Another consideration is that a shoe used for obstacle course racing must allow water to drain easily from the shoe as you are often required to run through water. There is nothing worse than running around in sloshing, heavy, water-soaked shoes. Due to the increased popularity of obstacle course racing, companies have now designed shoes specifically for the sport.

You will also need a good pair of road-running shoes as it is doubtful that you will do all your running on trails. There is nothing wrong with wearing trail shoes while running on the road; however, there are a few points to keep in mind. The first is that trail shoes are typically less cushioned than road shoes. So, if you are a heavier or high-mileage runner, this may be an issue. The second is that the traction on your trail shoe will wear down faster on the road. I prefer to have both a pair of road-running shoes and a pair of trail-running shoes.

This section was designed to give you the basic knowledge concerning the biomechanical rationale for shoe selection. Unless you have extensive experience in this area, I strongly recommend seeing a running shoe specialist, orthopedic specialist, or biomechanist in order to best determine the shoe that will work with your biomechanics.

Shoe Fit

There are key points to look for in a proper shoe fit. The first is that you should have a thumbs width between your big toe and the end of the shoe. This measurement will need to be conducted while standing. Next, with the shoes tied, the shoe should fit comfortably snug across the top of your foot (not tight). Finally, walk around to determine if the back of the shoe slips up and down on the heel of your foot. If the heel slides up and down excessively, the shoe is too large. Also keep in mind that shoes from different brands may fit differently. If one brand does not fit correctly on your foot, try another. Do not get caught in the trap of buying a brand or model just because you want it. Ultimately, the most important aspect is that the shoes fit comfortably on your feet. If they are not comfortable walking around the store, chances are strong that the shoes will be more uncomfortable on a run. Prior to running in your new shoes, I recommend going home and wearing the shoes around the house for a few hours to determine if they are truly comfortable. This way you can return the shoes for another size or brand if necessary. Some running stores will have treadmills set up in the store to allow you to walk or run in the store prior to purchasing the shoes.

Shoe Maintenance

Properly maintaining your shoes will prolong their life. It is important to keep your shoes dry and relatively clean in order to prevent premature breakdown. Your shoes are going to get soaking wet and muddy and there is no reason to try to avoid it. However, you do not want to store your shoes muddy and wet after use. Keeping them dry and clean becomes even more of an issue when you are running trails and obstacle course races. The easiest way to clean your shoes is with a hose. Just put the spray on high and wash all the mud off inside and out with the water and a scrub brush. Keep in mind that keeping your shoes clean and dry is not about keeping them looking nice. Instead, it is about prolonging the life of the shoe. If the shoe surface is caked in mud, it prevents airflow, which will mean a longer time for the shoe to dry. A wet, muddy environment is a great place for bacteria to grow and thrive. This will damage the material and result in a smell that will guarantee you won't have any running buddies. When cleaning your shoes, make sure to get all the rocks and mud out of the treads as well. Treads that are clogged will not grip as well on your next run, and the rocks that are imbedded within will continue to wear the treads during your run.

Once your shoes are clean, make sure that they dry as quickly as possible. First and foremost, do not put your shoes in the dryer as it will ruin them. In order to optimize drying time, loosen the laces, pull the tongue back, and remove the insert. This will allow more air to flow in. If it is a nice warm day, you can place your shoes outside to dry. Another method is to ball up newspaper and place it within the shoe to help absorb water. Wet shoes can also be set beside a dehumidifier or in front of a blowing fan to assist in the drying process.

It is an unfortunate fact that running shoes wear down and must be replaced somewhat frequently. Not only does the sole wear thin and lose traction, but the EVA material (the white cushioning material) becomes compressed and loses the ability to absorb ground reaction forces. The typical recommendations are to replace running shoes every 300 to 500 miles. The actual miles will vary due to the quality of the shoe, mass of the individual, intensity of the miles put on the shoes, and the conditions that the individual runs in. However, as long as the shoe is safe and comfortable there is no reason to purchase new shoes.

Where to Buy

Where to buy running shoes will depend a lot on your knowledge and ability. If you currently know your running biomechanics (in-line, overpronation, or supination) and the brand, style, and size of your preferred shoe, then you can save a substantial amount of money by ordering online. I typically try to find closeout deals on models that are a year or two old and spend about half the money in relation to buying the newest model at retail. The vast majority of the time, the only difference between a model that is one to two years older and the brand-new model is the color.

However, if you currently do not know the brand, style, and size of the shoe you need and have minimal knowledge on choosing the correct running shoe, I would advise visiting a specialized running store. Shopping at a running store that specializes in fitting running shoes will save you money in the long run. If you blindly buy a shoe online due to a lower price, it may or may not work for you. If the shoe does not work with your particular running biomechanics, then you just wasted money on a pair of shoes you cannot train in. Going to a reputable running store that provides gait analysis and shoe fit is highly recommended.

There is a difference between a store that sells running shoes and a true running store. A true running store will analyze your gait while walking and running, choose a group of shoes for you to try on, ensure proper fit and comfort, reanalyze again in the chosen shoes, and then make final recommendations. If the running store uses video analysis software, they may not analyze your walk and may instead go straight into analyzing your run. When conducting a visual analysis, without video analysis, it is sometimes helpful to observe an individual walking at slower speeds prior to having them run. However, this step is not necessary when using video analysis because the specialist can slow the video down and observe the kinematics of your run frame by frame. If you visit a store that carries running shoes and the staff does not take the time to analyze and fit you in the correct shoes, politely break away and visit another store. Local runners will typically be able to tell you which stores to visit and which to stay away from.

While you may be able to save money purchasing shoes online, there are benefits to buying shoes at a running-specialty store. The first involves immersing yourself in the community. Getting to know the running and OCR community will provide you with a wealth of knowledge concerning running, training, the sport of triathlon, and local races. The second is that by supporting your local running shop, they will continue to be around to support you and the local training and racing community.

CLOTHING

The most important aspects to consider concerning clothing and running are comfort and environment. Luckily when it comes to clothing for running, you do not need to spend a lot of money. While you can spend quite a bit on name brands, there really is no need, as an off-brand shirt made of the same material will perform just the same as a big-name brand. When purchasing running clothes, consider material, fit, and comfort.

Avoid running in 100-percent cotton shirts and shorts. Cotton is not breathable, will retain water, negatively impacts heat dissipation, and can chafe (cotton is rough against the skin). This becomes even more important during obstacle course races where you are periodically submerged in water. Instead choose material made from synthetic fibers (primarily polyester) that are specifically woven in a manner that allows moisture transfer from the skin and evaporation sweat to occur. Nylon is another synthetic fiber commonly used in athletic attire; however, it does not wick moisture away in the same manner as polyester and therefore does not have the same cooling affect. The difference between a poorly made synthetic-fiber shirt and a well-made synthetic-fiber shirt is the shape of the individual fibers and the alignment of the fiber. While you want to avoid 100 percent cotton, cotton blend is a good choice as it allows greater breathability, and it does not develop the same smell as all-synthetic gear.

Clothing should fit comfortably and not chafe during the run. The most common places for chafing are inner thighs, underarms, nipples, and bra area for females. Common causes of chafing are large or rough seams and rough, wet material repeatedly moving across the skin. Keep in mind that on long runs chafing can occur even when wearing the best clothing. To prevent chafing during long runs, use Band-Aids or an anti-chafing gel in the affected areas.

Females should consider wearing a sports bra in order to provide support and limit chafing while running. A sports bra differs from a normal bra in that it will typically fit comfortably snug, is made of synthetic material for wicking moisture, and has a band along the bottom to help hold it in place. Do not get hung up on looks; concentrate more on support and comfort.

In general, clothing for running in the summer should be breathable so that heat can be easily dissipated. Clothing should also be light in color so that it does not easily absorb heat. During the winter, clothing should be layered to wick moisture away from the skin and insulate against the cold. A common mistake is to overdress during the winter, causing the runner to overheat on a run.

HEART RATE MONITOR

It is vitally important to monitor and control workout intensity during training and heart rate is an excellent tool for monitoring intensity. While you can measure pulse rate with your fingers and a watch, it is not as accurate and convenient as using a heart rate monitor to measure heart rate. Proper use of a heart rate monitor will be covered later in this book.

A heart rate monitor consists of a transmitter and a receiver. The transmitter fits around the thoracic region just below the pectoralis major. When placing the transmitter below the chest, it is important to center the transmitter midline. The transmitter should be tight enough not to move around, but not so tight as to be uncomfortable. The transmitter should be wet and placed against the skin in order to pick up the electrical impulse of the heart contractions. The receiver acquires the signal from the transmitter and then displays heart rate. Traditionally the receiver has been worn on the wrist as a watch. However, you can now use a Bluetooth transmitter that connects to your smartphone, where you can record heart rate using various applications.

The heart rate monitor will have various functions that are useful for maintaining intensity and evaluating performance. Heart rate monitors vary in price based on function ($40 to over $300). An entry-level heart rate monitor that provides heart rate and time only will start at around $40. I recommend purchasing a heart rate monitor that at least has zone alarms. This will allow you to set alarms that sound when you go below (typically not a problem) or above (usually the problem) your training zone for the day. If you are going to train in a group, you need a heart rate monitor that is coded so that you do not pick up another triathlete's heart rate as you train.

For those athletes serious about training, I recommend purchasing an entry-level heart rate monitor that provides GPS data. These units are not inexpensive, but they are an extremely valuable training tool, providing not only heart rate but also GPS data. One of the unique benefits of this system is the ability to download both heart rate and GPS data after a workout for analysis. As a coach I find this feature invaluable. I can examine my athlete's heart rate in relation to alterations in grade, speed, and distance.

When choosing a heart rate monitor, there are other options you can consider as well, but these are the basics. One last thing to mention is that I have seen many athletes spend a lot of money on heart rate monitors but then never really use them. At that point, the heart rate monitor just becomes an expensive toy as opposed to a powerful training tool. Before purchasing an expensive heart rate monitor, seriously consider how you will integrate the system into your training program.

WORKOUT FACILITIES

The various obstacles that you will traverse during an obstacle course race will require the use of both muscular endurance and muscular strength. Due to those requirements, it is important that you have a workout facility that allows you to train for both. When choosing a workout facility, there are key aspects to consider. The first is whether they have all the necessary workout equipment you require for optimal training. There are some gyms that do not have free weights and others that may contain free weights only. Choose a gym with a mixture of free weights and machines that will allow you to accomplish your strength and conditioning goals. When choosing a gym, you also need to know what types of lifts are permitted. For example, some gyms do not allow deadlifts.

There are gyms that specialize in obstacle course racing and will have all the equipment you need for training. They will have overhead obstacles, walls, ropes, atlas stones, tires, and other various pieces of equipment that will allow you to focus on training for specific obstacles. Specialized OCR gyms will also be staffed with individuals who have a background in obstacle course racing. If you are lucky enough to have an OCR gym in your area, definitely give it a try.

It is also important to know the gym's operating hours in order to determine if it will fit within your schedule. I advise visiting the gym during the primary time slot that you plan on working out so you can determine if it is busy at that particular time. While you are visiting, make sure to ask when the high-traffic times are. High-traffic times typically extend your workout length as there may be longer wait times on equipment.

If you are serious about strength and conditioning and have the available space, you may want to consider building a home gym. This makes your strength and conditioning workouts more convenient. Considering the average cost of a gym membership is about $600 per year (this is a very conservative figure and will vary greatly by area), it may be a better idea to invest the money in a home gym. Building a home gym is not as expensive as you may think. I buy greater than 90 percent of my equipment secondhand, as many people buy workout equipment, never use it, and then sell it at a significantly reduced rate. If you buy used equipment, always examine it for any defects. As I have been physically active my entire life and plan on continuing for the remainder of my life, a home gym is a good investment for me. I also live in the country and the closest gym is 25 minutes away. You will need to decide if a home gym is a good investment for you.

Very few gyms have obstacles available for you to train on. You may want to consider building a small course in your backyard. This would allow you to train for overhead obstacles, rope climbs, wall climbs, etc., at home. There are many different design options you can find online. You should be able to find ideas that will fit within your given training space and budget. Keep in mind that your setup does not have to be elaborate or expensive to be effective.

If you decide to develop a home gym, you may also want to consider flooring. I divided my gym into a weight-training area and a conditioning area. On the weight-training side, I use black horse mats for the floor as they are durable and hard enough for the weights, yet provide some cushioning. Horse mats are also much less expensive per square foot than gym flooring of the same durability. The downside of horse mats is that you will typically need to let them air out in your garage prior to putting them in the house due to the rubber smell that is common. Once they air out, the smell goes away. On the conditioning side of my gym, I use a martial arts puzzle-type mat that is durable, provides cushioning, and is nonslip. If you choose to go this route, do not buy the inexpensive puzzle mats you find in common retail stores. These mats are not durable and will not last very long. Do not lift free weights on the conditioning mats as they will damage the mat.

2

BASIC TRAINING PRINCIPLES, PHYSIOLOGY, AND PSYCHOLOGY

This chapter provides the necessary background knowledge on training principles, physiology, and psychology required for you to better determine how you will plan and implement your training program for obstacle course racing (OCR). In order to create and adhere to a quality training program, it is important to understand how your body will respond to the stress applied during training and competition. The body responds to stress in very specific ways, which has allowed for the development of training principles that can be directly applied to your training program with predictable outcomes. Gaining an understanding of these basic principles will help you to make better training choices.

BASIC TRAINING PRINCIPLES

Training Adaptations

Training adaptations are how the body responds to the applied training stimulus over time. These adaptations can either be positive or negative depending on the type, volume, and intensity of the training stimulus. The goal of proper training is to manipulate these three factors in order to elicit a physiological response that will lead to positive training adaptations and increased OCR performance. Incorrectly manipulating these factors can lead to improper physiological adaptations and, therefore, no alterations to performance. Additionally, improper training can lead to negative adaptations and subsequent decreases in performance.

Individual Differences

The principle of individual differences states that not every individual responds to the same training stimulus in the same manner. For example, some recover quicker and can handle a higher training volume or intensity. Others may require longer recovery periods and therefore cannot handle higher volumes or frequent high-intensity bouts of training. It is important to individualize your training program so that you optimize training volume and recovery time.

While most individuals are born with approximately 50 percent slow twitch muscle fibers (good for endurance) and 50 percent fast twitch (good for anaerobic exercise), some are born with a greater percentage of slow twitch or fast twitch fibers. Therefore, some individuals will be predisposed to greater improvements in endurance while others will be predisposed to greater improvements in anaerobic activity, strength, and power. Obstacle course racing is an endurance sport filled with events that require anaerobic capacity, muscular endurance, muscular strength, and muscular power.

Current training status is also an obvious factor. Those who have been training longer will be able to handle greater volume and intensity than beginning racers. If you are new to OCR, you will need to start off slowly, learn proper technique, and maintain consistency.

Athletes and coaches will often overlook individual differences and use a generic boxed training program that does not vary based on individual progression and can often hinder progress by delaying it. Conversely, if the training program is too strenuous, it can lead to overtraining and burnout. That said, it is okay to use a boxed training program to begin with, but adjustments to volume and intensity need to be made based on your response to that program.

Progressive Overload

The progressive overload principle states that the training stimulus needs to be continuously increased, allowing for adequate recovery between bouts, so that performance will improve. You can increase stimulus by either increasing volume or intensity. For the endurance portion of your training, volume is increased by either increasing duration (distance or time) of training sessions or frequency (number of training sessions). Intensity is altered by changing how hard the workout session is conducted. Volume should always be increased prior to increasing intensity. Make sure you can complete the distance before focusing on how fast you can complete it. For beginners, increasing intensity prior to increasing volume also increases the risk of injury. For muscular endurance and muscular strength, volume is increased by increasing the number of exercises, the number of sets, or the number of repetitions. Intensity is increased by increasing resistance (weight).

Principle of Hard and Easy

The hard–easy principle states that you cannot train hard every day and instead must alternate hard and easy days to optimize training adaptations. While this principle does oversimplify the problem, it does work, especially in the development of a training program for obstacle course racing. When designing a workout program, it is important to alternate your hard and easy days so that you will have ample time for recovery. Too many hard days in a row will result in overtraining due to lack of recovery between bouts. Examining intensity is one way to determine your hard and easy days. Interval sessions are examples of hard days, whereas runs below anaerobic threshold would be considered easy days. Keep in mind that your long run of the week is also considered a hard day, even though it is below threshold. Training for OCR has an extra challenge in that you will have to also work muscular endurance and muscular strength training into your program.

Recovery

Too often racers focus so much on training that they forget one of the most important components of increasing performance: recovery. Training is catabolic (meaning that molecules are broken down into smaller constituents) in nature, ultimately resulting in protein synthesis after the training bout. To optimize the body's response to the training stimuli, make sure that adequate recovery occurs between bouts.

Alternate hard and easy days to optimize recovery. It is important to monitor intensity so that you do not train too hard too often. This is a common mistake made by most racers. During recovery it is also important to focus on recovery nutrition in order to refuel and optimize protein synthesis. Also important is to maintain a minimum of eight hours of good sleep every night.

Overtraining

One of the most common threats to OCR performance is overtraining. In most cases, a racer will compete better 10 percent undertrained than 1 percent overtrained. To optimize performance, racers continually walk the line of optimal performance and overtraining. Overtraining occurs when adequate recovery is not allowed between bouts and is often the result of a sudden increase in volume and/or intensity or an accumulation of a small imbalance of recovery and training.

As an obstacle course racer, be aware of how your body responds to training and know the signs and symptoms of overtraining. Common signs for overtraining include:

- Multiple sessions of decreased performance. One bad day does not necessarily indicate overtraining. However, multiple days of decreased performance does indicate overtraining.
- Feeling of constant fatigue.
- Poor attitude.
- A feeling of dread about training.
- Abnormal sleeping patterns.
- An increase in resting heart rate measured on multiple days. An increase on one day may indicate that you have not recovered from the previous day's workout or that you may be dehydrated. However, if the increase in resting heart rate persists over multiple days, it is a strong indicator of overtraining.
- Consistent overuse injuries.
- Chronic illness due to a lowered immune response.
- Abrupt changes in body composition.

Specificity of Training

Training adaptations are specific to the training stimulus applied. In simpler terms, train the body in the manner in which you would like for it to adapt. For example, cycling is a great endurance sport, but you do not cycle during an obstacle course race. Therefore, when training for OCR it would not make sense for you to cycle and spend very little time running as running is specific to obstacle course racing. Obstacle course races are held on trails, and therefore you should train on trails. Trail running is subtly different than road running and requires a specific set of skills. Learning how to pace over rough terrain, navigate the quickest and safest path on the trail, and handle the steep up and down sections of a course requires practice.

You will also want to train specifically for the obstacles that you will be completing in competition. While obstacles do vary from race to race, they all share a common core. For example, you know there will be a lot of overhead obstacles (rings, dial rods, bars, etc.), and therefore you will need to train for those obstacles. The common obstacles found in OCR and how to train for them will be discussed in the following chapter.

Detraining

Detraining occurs when you decrease or remove the training stimulus, which leads to a decrease in performance and the loss of training adaptations over time. Put quite simply, if you do not use it, you lose it. Common reasons for detraining include injury, illness, and improper off-season training. Typically detraining begins after two weeks of inactivity. This does not mean that you lose all adaptations after two weeks of no training. It just means that there is a slight measurable difference after that amount of time. However, I have seen people who were overtrained improve after two weeks of recovery.

Detraining is one of the biggest fears of most OCR athletes, which often leads to overtraining. Many racers believe that taking a few days off from training will negatively impact performance. However, taking a couple days off on occasion will not hurt your performance and could, in fact, be beneficial if you are overtrained. However, do not use the fear of overtraining as an excuse to take multiple days off on a regular basis.

If you must scale down or completely stop training due to illness or injury, it will not take too long to get back to where you left off. When returning to training, do not try to start at the same volume and intensity where you left off. Instead, start off slowly and work your way back. Start by increasing volume first, and then increase intensity. Coming back too quickly can lead to injury and further delays in training. This is especially true if the time off from training occurred due to injury.

Consistency

Your training plan should be well laid out and consistent in terms of frequency of training. One of the common mistakes that beginners make is to train haphazardly; they might train four days a week for a couple weeks, then two days the following week, and then one day a week for the next couple weeks. In this scenario, increases in performance would be unlikely or minimal at best.

Inconsistent training may also lead to injury. Trying to automatically pick up where you left off in training places too much stress on the body. For the best gains and to reduce the risk of injury, follow your training program. If life gets in the way, which it does, then alter your training program to minimize the impact.

Frequency

Frequency is defined as how often you train. This can be measured in days or in the number of training sessions. Beginning OCR athletes should train a minimum of three to four days per week, with a day off or an easy day between workouts. This method allows you to train harder on workout days and then recover prior to your next workout. Training only three or four days per week will be just enough to get you across the finish line; however, it will not get you to the finish line quickly.

To determine frequency of your workouts, first consider your current fitness level. As a beginner, you should start on the lower end and work your way up. Also consider time management. Family, work, school, and other commitments must be considered when developing a training schedule. Find a way to balance all aspects of your life so that you are ultimately happy. For me, family will always come first, then work, then training.

Duration

Duration is the length of your training session, which will be determined by the goal of that session. For endurance training, the duration will be determined by the desired intensity for that session. Duration and intensity are inversely related, meaning that as one goes up, the other must go down. You cannot run a 10k race at the same pace you would a 5k race. As the distance increases, the intensity will decrease. You can determine the length of your endurance training sessions by specifying a time limit or a specific distance. For running, I usually prefer distance over time because it allows for a more precise measure. If the goal for the day is a mid-distance run at an easy pace, it makes more sense to state that you will run for 3 to 6 miles (depending on your current fitness level) at a heart rate that is equal to your easy training zone, and then mark the time when you are finished. This method will give you more precise measures as opposed to running for a specific time period. However, you must keep in mind that obstacle course races are held on trails, and due to the varying nature of trails, a relatively flat 3-mile trail will take much less time in relation to a 3-mile trail with a lot of climbing. You should be able to complete the distance of your planned race prior to race day to ensure that you have an enjoyable race.

Duration for your muscular endurance and strength training will be determined by the number of exercises, number of sets, and number of repetitions. First determine how many exercises you wish to conduct during your training session, and then determine the number of sets per exercise. Next, decide the number of repetitions per exercise. To increase muscular endurance, you will typically be using body weight management skills (pull-ups, push-ups, crunches, etc.), and you will increase the number of repetitions per set in order to increase duration. When working to improve muscular strength and muscular endurance, keep your repetitions between 8 and 15 per exercise.

Intensity

Intensity is the "how hard" of training, and it is extremely important to properly manipulate in order for appropriate training adaptations to occur. The hard-easy principle, mentioned previously, is one method of addressing training intensity. There will be weeks when you will have more than one hard day in a row, but they must be purposeful and planned carefully.

For endurance training, intensity levels can be categorized into three basic levels: below anaerobic threshold, at anaerobic threshold, and above anaerobic threshold. When training or racing, you will be at one of these three physiological intensities. Below threshold intensities involve workouts that are below race pace—active recovery training, easy mid-distance training, and long, slow distance. At-threshold training consists of race pace and tempo work (short tempo work may actually be above threshold). Above-threshold training involves interval and overreaching training. Knowing and understanding intensity levels helps you to better plan a training regimen that ensures you do not overtrain. How to properly determine intensity levels for endurance training will be discussed in the next chapter.

Intensity for muscular strength and endurance is determined by the resistance you use with weight training, which is determined by the number of sets desired or by the percentage of your one repetition max (1RM). I usually recommend avoiding 1RMs with many athletes as it adds a small degree of unnecessary risk. With certain sports and a certain level of athletes, I do recommend using 1RMs to monitor progress. However, for the majority of people reading this book, it will be unnecessary as in all situations you will adjust the weight as necessary to maintain the desired repetitions per set. If your goal is to stay between 8 and 15 repetitions for three sets, you will pick a weight that allows you to stay between 8 and 15 repetitions for all three sets.

Warming Up

It is important to warm up prior to exercise in order to optimize performance and decrease the risk of injury. While a direct link between a warm-up and a decreased risk of injury has yet to be determined, there is a strong correlation between injury rates and lack of a warm-up. When examining sport performance, warming up facilitates three important aspects. First, the warm-up will redirect blood flow to working muscles. Second, there will be an increase in cardiac output due to an increase in both heart rate and stroke volume. And third, muscle temperature will increase, which improves muscular performance. It typically takes about two minutes to sufficiently increase cardiac output, increase muscle temperature, and redirect blood flow to the point that oxygen supply is equivalent to demand in the working muscles. All of these factors will result in increased performance.

A warm-up for OCR should consist of about 5 minutes of easy jogging, followed by about 5 to 10 minutes of stretching, and then finished off with another bout of running, adding in some upper-body work (push-ups, pull-ups, etc.) during the run. Be sure to stretch your upper body as well as your lower. If it is a low-intensity training day, such as a recovery run, then you can go right into the run after the brief stretching. If it is a hard training day (tempo work or intervals) or a race, then adjust the second warm-up run accordingly. When warming up for a race, the second warm-up run should consist of short intervals that take you to the race pace of the distance you are racing for that particular event. If it is a race day, make sure to time your warm-up so that you finish at the start line in time to line up for your race.

Cooling Down

Conducting a cool-down after a workout is an important part of your training program. An active cool-down will slowly bring your heart rate down and prevent blood from pooling in your legs. If you suddenly stop after a hard bout of exercise and blood pools in your legs, it could result in dizziness. While dizziness under these conditions is not overly common, it is not uncommon. As you run during an active recovery cool-down, the muscle pump in the legs will assist with blood return to the heart, preventing the blood from pooling in the legs. An active cool-down will also help clear blood lactate after high-intensity bouts. A cool-down will not prevent the development of a delayed onset of muscle soreness, however.

A cool-down should consist of 5 to 15 minutes of easy running followed by 10 to 15 minutes of stretching. The harder the workout, the longer the cool-down should be. Cool-down after a recovery run should take much less time than cool-down after an interval session.

Delayed Onset of Muscle Soreness

If you work out, it is inevitable that you will experience delayed onset of muscle soreness (DOMS). This is the pain you feel the day after a workout. It will typically last one to three days, depending on the extent of the muscular damage. In severe cases, DOMS can last much longer. There is a common misconception that DOMS occurs due to a buildup of lactic acid. However, this is not the case. DOMS occurs due to tiny tears in muscle tissue during eccentric contractions (when muscle lengthens during the contraction). Edema then develops due to the damage, and as the swelling continues, pressure builds up, pushing on nerve endings and resulting in pain.

BASIC PHYSIOLOGY

Physiology Overview

In order to correctly apply training principles for optimal performance, it is important to have a basic understanding of physiology as it applies to sport. This understanding will help you to determine the type of training stimulus that will best lead to adaptations for increased performance in obstacle course racing. There are many "experts" that claim to have the best method for increased performance. Some of these methods work well, but some of the proposed methods are unsubstantiated fads that will not lead to increased performance and in some cases lead to a decrease in performance. The more informed you are on the subject, the better you will be able to make an educated decision.

Knowledge of physiology as it is applied to sport performance will also help you determine if your body is correctly adapting to the applied training stimulus. If you understand the physiological adaptations that should occur, then you can better gauge the degree to which your training program elicits these changes.

The key to understanding physiology comes from two terms driven into my head through eight years of school (undergrad through Ph.D., not eight years of undergrad!): form and function. Every element of the body is formed for specific function. Adaptations, occurring due to training, may even slightly alter form in order to improve function. Understanding the function of a system, organ, hormone, substrate, or enzyme will allow you to determine the effect of each on human performance. The first part of this section will cover basic physiology in order to provide a foundation that will help you to grasp the physiological adaptations that occur due to endurance training.

Cardiorespiratory Endurance

The cardiorespiratory system is comprised of the cardiovascular system and the respiratory system. The cardiovascular system is comprised of the heart and blood vessels and is responsible for the movement of blood through the body. Movement of blood through the body is vital as it is responsible for transporting oxygen, glucose, free fatty acids, hormones, and other key substrates to the working muscle. Equally important are the byproducts that blood carries away from the working tissue (carbon dioxide and lactate).

The respiratory system is comprised of air passages and lungs and is responsible for the transport and diffusion of gasses. Air moves through the air passageways, bringing in vital oxygen to the lungs where it is diffused across the respiratory membrane and into the lungs. Carbon dioxide crosses the respiratory membrane into the lungs and then is exhaled into the atmosphere.

The cardiorespiratory system is key during endurance performance and many times will limit performance based on the individual's current fitness level. There are adaptations that occur due to endurance training that greatly improve the body's ability to transport blood and oxygen. These adaptations will be discussed later in this chapter.

Heart

The heart is a specialized muscle (myocardium) designed to pump blood through the body. The heart differs from other muscles in that it is the most oxidative muscle in the body; it is designed to conduct the electrical impulse rapidly, and the signal for contraction originates in the muscle (sinoatrial node). The heart consists of four chambers (left and right atria and left and right ventricles). Pulmonary circulation (right atrium and ventricle) is designed to pump oxygen-poor blood returning from the body into the lungs. Systemic circulation (left atrium and ventricle) is designed to pump oxygen-rich blood to the body.

I will make a long, complicated story short. Oxygen-poor blood returns to the right side of the heart and then is pumped to the lungs where CO_2 is released from the blood and O_2 is picked up. The oxygen-rich blood then travels to the left side of the heart where it is pumped out to the body. The blood then travels through smaller and smaller arteries until it reaches arterioles and then capillaries at the tissue. This is where oxygen, nutrients, water, carbon dioxide, and other byproducts are transported to and from the tissue. As the capillaries leave the tissue, they connect to venules and then veins before returning to the heart.

The heart is not strong enough to pump blood down through the body and then back up toward the heart against gravity from the lower extremities. There are mechanisms in place that assist with blood return to the heart. The first is called the muscle pump. Muscles in the leg contract rhythmically, causing blood to be pushed upward during the contraction phase. When the muscles relax, one-way valves in the veins prevent the blood from flowing back down. The second method is the respiratory pump. Changes in thoracic pressure due to breathing aid in blood return to the heart.

The muscle pump is one of the reasons that an active cool-down is beneficial after a high-intensity workout. As you are walking or jogging during your active recovery, the muscles in the legs are contracting forcefully and rhythmically, pushing blood back toward the heart with every contraction. This prevents pooling of blood in the lower extremities after a workout.

Cardiac Output

Cardiac output is the volume of blood pumped per minute and is a product of stroke volume and heart rate ($Q = SV \times HR$). Stroke volume is the volume of blood pumped from the left ventricle in each beat, and heart rate is defined as the number of times the heart beats each minute. Cardiac output responds to exercise by increasing linearly with increases in intensity until max intensity is reached. Heart rate also increases linearly with an increase in intensity. Stroke volume can nearly double from resting but will only increase to about 50 percent of maximal intensity, and then it levels off. So after about 50 percent of max intensity, all increases in cardiac output will come primarily from heart rate only.

Autoregulation of Blood Flow

Autoregulation of blood flow concerns the redirection of blood flow based on tissue need. Blood flow is redirected by altering blood vessel diameter through vasoconstriction and vasodilatation. As we move from a resting state to an exercising state, metabolism substantially increases. Going for an easy run can increase metabolism by six to nine times above resting levels. Because the metabolic demand of the working muscles increases substantially during exercise, a greater amount of blood flow must be sent to the working muscle to increase the delivery of oxygen and nutrients. During exercise, blood flow is redirected to the working muscles, skin (for cooling), heart, and brain and reduced in areas where it is less needed, such as the digestive system and kidneys. During rest, approximately 20 percent of blood flow travels to the muscles. During exercise, as much as 80 percent of blood flow can be redirected to muscles.

Understanding this concept is vital for a complete understanding of the body's response to exercise. For example, autoregulation of blood flow explains the body's response to exercise after eating. You have probably eaten a meal and then exercised at some point in your life. Even if you are not completely miserable exercising right after a meal, the experience is never as comfortable as you would like it to be and your performance is subpar. The reason behind this is that your digestive system is in direct competition with the working muscles for blood flow. Due to fight or flight, the sympathetic response will win out over the parasympathetic response and greater blood flow will go to the muscles. However, a greater amount of blood will be redirected to the digestive system compared to exercising without prior food consumption. Because of the redirection of blood flow to the digestive system, your performance will decrease and your stomach may become upset.

When exercising in the heat, a greater amount of blood flow will be redirected to the skin for cooling than if you were training in a thermo-neutral environment. Dissipating heat is vital for survival and will take priority over blood flow to muscles. Due to this, performance decreases in a hot environment.

Blood

Blood is made up of around 55 percent plasma, 45 percent red blood cells (erythrocytes), and less than 1 percent white blood cells (leukocytes) and platelets. Hematocrit, the ratio of red blood cells in relation to whole blood, is used to measure the particular makeup of an individual's blood. The average hematocrit for a male is around 45, and for a female it is around 42.

Blood plays five major roles: transportation, heat transfer, acid base balance, coagulation, and immune response. While all five are important, we typically concentrate on the first three in exercise physiology as they have the greatest impact on performance. Each red blood cell contains a very large volume of hemoglobin molecules, which are responsible for the transportation of oxygen. Hemoglobin is comprised of a globin protein and a heme ring. The heme ring contains four iron molecules, and each of these iron molecules can bind one oxygen. This is why those who suffer from iron deficiency feel fatigued and have difficulty exercising.

Blood is extremely important when it comes to heat dissipation. Water makes up about 90 percent of plasma, which is why plasma is an excellent mechanism for heat transfer. Heat is transferred from the core and the working muscles to the blood where it is dissipated at the skin's surface. Plasma is also important for cooling as it provides sweat for evaporation through the skin; this statement is oversimplified as plasma moving from the blood vessels to the interstitial space to the skin is a complicated process.

It is vital that the acid base balance (pH) is maintained in order for the body to correctly function. Keep in mind that pH levels differ depending on the location in the body. The average muscle pH is about 7.1, whereas the average blood pH is around 7.4. It does not take a large drop in pH before physiological systems are affected. A drop in muscle pH from 7.1 to 6.9 will begin to negatively impact energy systems, leading to a decrease in performance. Blood helps maintain pH through the use of chemical buffers.

Gas Exchange

Endurance athletes need to be concerned with gas exchange in the lungs and tissue (primarily muscle). Henry's law states that gas dissolves in liquids because of three factors: partial pressure of the individual gas, solubility of a specific gas in a specific fluid, and temperature. While all three affect how gases dissolve in liquid, partial pressure is the main driving force behind gas exchange in the body. The types of fluids and gases do not alter in the human body. However, temperatures do, and this change affects the oxyhemaglobin disassociation curve, but the main driving force is the partial pressure of each gas.

To understand the importance of partial pressure, it is important to know Dalton's law: the sum of each individual pressure of each individual gas is equivalent to the total pressure of the mixture of gases. At sea level the atmospheric pressure is equivalent to 760 mmHg, which gives you the total pressure of the mixture of gases (air). What becomes important for understanding gas exchange is the partial pressure of each individual gas in the mixture. Oxygen makes up 20.93 percent of the total mixture, resulting in a partial pressure of oxygen (PO_2) equal to 159 mmHg. Carbon dioxide makes up .03 percent of the total mixture, resulting in a partial pressure of carbon dioxide (PCO_2) of .2 mmHg. Lastly, nitrogen accounts for 79.04 percent of the total mixture, resulting in a partial pressure of nitrogen (PN_2) of 600.7 mmHg. One thing to keep in mind is that atmospheric pressure alters as you leave sea level. If you were to leave sea level and travel to the top of Mt. Evans in Colorado, the atmospheric pressure would decrease to around 460 mmHg. Because the atmospheric pressure decreases and there are no alterations to the percentage of each individual gas, the partial pressure of each gas will decrease.

The alveoli are air sacs at the end of air tubes located in the lungs, which are responsible for oxygen and carbon dioxide exchange. Gas exchange occurs across the respiratory membrane, which lies between the alveoli and the capillaries. While the PO_2 in the atmosphere at sea level is equivalent to 159 mmHg, the PO_2 will decrease to around 105 mmHg in the alveoli. At rest, oxygen-poor blood will return to the lungs at a PO_2 of around 40 mmHg. The pressure differential of 60 mmHg will cause oxygen to move from the alveoli to the capillaries. Because alveolar PO_2 is maintained at 105 mmHg (it is not a closed system), oxygenated blood will leave the heart at a PO_2 of around 100 mmHg.

The alveoli PCO_2 remains at a constant 40 mmHg. The PCO_2 of blood returning to the heart will be approximately 46 mmHg. While the pressure differential is not as large compared to oxygen, carbon dioxide diffuses at a much greater rate across the respiratory membrane than oxygen. Therefore, the gradient does not have to be as large.

Muscle

Skeletal muscle originates and inserts on bone and crosses at least one joint. Therefore, the primary purpose of skeletal muscle is human movement. There are over 600 muscles in the human body, and it is important that you be able to name and identify all of them (just kidding). But it is important that you learn the primary muscles used in OCR in order to ensure proper strengthening and flexibility of those muscles.

Each skeletal muscle is composed of numerous muscle fibers. These muscle fibers are classified by characteristics and divided into slow twitch (type I) and fast twitch (type II with subcategories of IIa, IIx, and recently discovered IIb) muscle fibers. Slow twitch fibers are highly oxidative, fatigue resistant, and optimal for endurance performance. Type II, fast twitch, fibers are larger than intermediate and slow twitch fibers, and are more glycolytic, produce more force, and are good for events that require anaerobic energetics, strength, and power. These fibers contract and relax very quickly, but fatigue easily, which means they are great for initiating a sprint for the finish line.

Intermediate fibers are technically classified as a fast twitch fiber but fall between fast twitch and slow twitch. The reason IIa is classified as fast twitch is that it is slightly more glycolytic as opposed to oxidative. While you cannot alter fiber type through training, you can increase metabolic capabilities with intense training. If you were to train seriously for power, strength, or anaerobic performance, then intermediate fibers would shift toward greater glycolytic characteristics. If you were to train seriously for endurance performance, then oxidative processes would increase. Intermediate fibers will never be as oxidative as slow twitch fibers or as glycolytic as fast twitch fibers; the properties will shift toward type of training. Intermediate fibers recruitment will increase as intensity increases

Slow twitch fibers are of the utmost importance for OCR competitors as they are primarily oxidative muscle fibers. Slow twitch fibers do not activate as quickly as fast twitch and do not produce as much force. However, they are slow to fatigue and ideal for endurance activities.

Distribution of muscle fiber type is genetic, and most people are born with 50 percent slow twitch and 50 percent fast twitch (including intermediate). Some individuals are born with a greater amount of one type of fiber or another. Elite-level endurance athletes will typically possess up to around 80 percent slow twitch fibers, whereas an elite-level Olympic lifter can have around 65 percent fast twitch fibers. The predominate theory is that muscle fiber types cannot change from one type to another through training. Muscle fiber distribution can be determined through a muscle biopsy, which is expensive and painful, and therefore typically not recommended.

Muscle fibers are arranged in functional groups called motor units. Each motor unit consists of only one type of muscle fiber and is innervated by a motor neuron. A slow twitch motor unit will have a small amount of muscle fibers, 10–180, and a fast twitch motor unit will contain anywhere from 300 to 800 muscle fibers. The number of motor units in a muscle is highly dependent on the size of the muscle. The numbers range from around 100 in a small muscle to over 1,500 in a larger muscle.

It is important to understand how motor units function as well as how they are recruited to contract. When the signal to contract travels down the motor neuron to the muscle fibers of the motor unit, all muscle fibers in that unit will contract. This is known as the all-or-none response. It is like a light switch; it is either on or off. However, not all the motor units in a muscle will contract during a task. We recruit only those motor units necessary to accomplish the task at hand.

Motor units are recruited in a specific pattern based on the size of the motor unit. Due to this, slow twitch motor units are recruited first, followed by intermediate fibers, and then fast twitch fibers. Recruitment is designed for optimal economy. When performing any task, you will recruit only the minimum amount of motor units to accomplish the task; primarily slow twitch fibers. The higher the intensity, the more intermediate and fast twitch fibers will be recruited. As these fibers are not very oxidative, you will fatigue sooner at higher intensities. Through training, neuromuscular recruitment patterns alter, allowing you to become more proficient at the skill. This adaptation improves economy and ultimately performance.

Energy Systems

Energy is required in order for human movement to occur. Competing in OCR requires repetitive muscle contractions and significant increases in metabolism. As you move from resting to exercise, metabolism increases exponentially. Going from resting metabolism to an easy run increases energy requirements six to nine times that of resting requirements.

Humans derive energy from the ingestion of food. There are three primary sources for energy: lipids, carbohydrates, and proteins. The two main sources used for energy during exercise are lipids and carbohydrates. With the exception of extreme situations (starvation), protein will never provide a substantial source of energy. The main job of protein involves anabolic processes in the body. Carbohydrates are stored as glycogen in the muscles and liver and transported in the blood as glucose. Glycogen stores are limited to around 2,000 kCals. Lipids are stored as triacylglycerol (commonly referred to as triglycerides) in muscle and adipose tissue (under the skin and around organs). Storage of lipids varies greatly among individuals, with the average being 60,000 to 80,000 kCals. Naturally the volume of stored lipids can vary greatly as well. Excess protein is not stored in the body. Regardless of the source, all ingested food must be converted to adenosine triphosphate (ATP) in order for it to be utilized as fuel in the human body.

Energy systems are frequently categorized into aerobic and anaerobic systems. Aerobic systems are those systems that require oxygen for the metabolic processes to occur, and anaerobic systems are those that do not require oxygen for metabolic processes to occur. Under each of those broad categories are specific energy systems. There are four basic energy systems that provide ATP for human movement. It is important to understand each of these energy systems because it will affect training and your choice of nutrition.

Stored ATP

The first system is stored ATP in the muscles. While commonly classified as a system, stored ATP is more of a source than an actual system. Stores are limited, and therefore reliance on this system as a major energy source is also limited. Stored ATP will only provide energy for about two to three seconds before stores are depleted. Energy for the muscle contraction is provided when a phosphate is cleaved from ATP, leaving adenosine diphosphate (ADP) and a phosphate. This process does not require oxygen and provides energy quickly for immediate contraction. The remaining three energy systems are methods of producing ATP for energy. Once ATP is generated through these systems, a phosphate must be cleaved off to release the energy for muscle contraction.

ATP-PCr System

The second system is the ATP-PC$_r$ system. Phosphocreatine (PC$_r$) is stored in the muscle and is key in producing ATP. During this process, a phosphate is cleaved from PC$_r$ and donated to an ADP in order to form ATP. The ATP-PC$_r$ system is limited by PC$_r$ stores in the muscle and can only function as a major energy system for about 10 to 15 seconds. This system is anaerobic in nature and does not require oxygen to function. It takes about two minutes of recovery for PC$_r$ stores to replenish. This is a key consideration when planning rest intervals during resistance training.

Anaerobic Glycolysis

The next energy system is anaerobic glycolysis, which provides ATP through the catabolism of glucose and glycogen. This process does not require oxygen and can provide energy for up to 1.5 to 2 minutes. Anaerobic glycolysis produces two to three ATP per glucose or glycogen molecule. A decrease in pH is the limiting factor for energy production during anaerobic glycolysis. Muscle pH will decrease due to the hydrogen buildup that occurs during glycolysis. Glycolysis is a complex chemical process that stops at the creation of pyruvate. During anaerobic glycolysis two hydrogen bind with pyruvate to form lactic acid, which in turn will lose one hydrogen, becoming lactate. Lactic acid production is based on intensity level, which determines the speed of glycolysis and oxygen availability for metabolism.

Lactic acid is often considered as bad. However, this assumption is not correct as lactic acid is formed in order to decrease acidity. As mentioned previously, pyruvate picks up the excess hydrogen to decrease acidity. This binding is only temporary, and lactic acid releases the hydrogen ions and is converted into lactate (a salt molecule). Lactic acid itself is not the problem; instead it is the buildup of hydrogen. Hydrogen ions greatly increase acidity and will interfere with muscle contraction. The pain felt during high-intensity exercise, such as intervals, is the body's mechanism to signal you to slow down or come to a stop. Upon completion of exercise, lactic acid will be converted back into fuel through specific pathways and therefore should not be considered a waste product. Lastly, lactic acid is not responsible for delayed onset of muscle soreness.

Oxidative Phosphorylation

The first three systems provide energy quickly and without oxygen, and you will draw upon these energy systems periodically throughout the race. An obstacle course race is primarily an endurance event with short anaerobic bouts throughout. Most obstacles will require the use of anaerobic processes as many require muscular endurance or muscular strength.

As even the shortest obstacle course race will last longer than two minutes, the first three energy systems will not be used as the primary energy source, when looking at the race as a whole. Instead, oxidative phosphorylation will be used as the primary energy system for activity lasting longer than two minutes. Oxidative phosphorylation, as the name suggests, relies on oxygen for ATP production. There are two major pathways for energy production that fall under oxidative phosphorylation: the oxidation of carbohydrates and the oxidation of lipids. Duration and intensity will determine reliance on carbohydrates and lipids. Longer duration and lower intensity training will rely heavily on the oxidation of lipids, and higher intensity, shorter duration training will rely more heavily on the oxidation of carbohydrates. Typically, you will be using 80–100 percent carbohydrates at race pace during competition. During a recovery ride, you will be utilizing 60–80 percent lipids.

The first pathway under oxidative phosphorylation is the oxidation of carbohydrates, which produces ATP through the catabolism of glucose and glycogen. This process is often termed "aerobic glycolysis." The steps in aerobic glycolysis are the same as those used in anaerobic glycolysis. The main difference is that instead of pyruvate being converted to lactic acid, it is converted to acetyl-CoA, which moves on to the Krebs cycle (citric acid cycle) for ATP production. Aerobic glycolysis produces 36 to 39 ATP from one molecule of glucose or glycogen. The limiting factor for oxidation of carbohydrates is the amount of stored glycogen. As mentioned previously, the average stores of glycogen are equivalent to about 2,000 kCals. A runner will use approximately 100 kCals of glycogen per mile during a marathon. By mile 20 the runner would have utilized the 2,000 kCals of stored glycogen. Once glycogen stores are depleted, fatigue sets in.

The second pathway involves the oxidation of lipids. This process requires more oxygen, more chemical processes, and more time. However, ATP production is much greater with the oxidation of lipids. One triacylglycerol will produce approximately 460 ATP. With 60,000 to 80,000 kCals of lipids stored in the body, it would be impossible to completely deplete them during exercise. When fatigue occurs due to limitations of oxidative phosphorylation, it occurs due to depletion of glycogen stores.

Measurement of the Body's Ability to Deliver Oxygen ($VO_{2\,max}$)

Obstacle course racing is an endurance sport, and an individual's ability to perform is highly dependent on the athlete's ability to transport and utilize oxygen. There is a very strong correlation between an athlete's oxidative capacity and their performance during endurance events. Due to this, it has become common practice to test an endurance athlete's $VO_{2\,max}$ in order to determine current fitness level. $VO_{2\,max}$ is the body's maximal ability to deliver oxygen to the working muscles and the muscles' ability to use that oxygen to produce energy for movement. As $VO_{2\,max}$ increases with training, so too will endurance performance.

$VO_{2\,max}$ can be increased through proper training. The adaptations that occur due to endurance training are designed to increase oxygen transport and utilization. So as training increases, $VO_{2\,max}$ increases, and so too does performance. The extent to which $VO_{2\,max}$ can be increased through training is highly dependent on genetics; while everyone can increase $VO_{2\,max}$, improvements are limited by a predetermined genetic ceiling.

$VO_{2\,max}$ can be expressed in absolute (l/m) or relative (ml/kg/min) terms. Expressing $VO_{2\,max}$ through relative terms is the preferred method as it more accurately represents endurance performance relative to body mass: milliliters of oxygen consumed per kilogram of body mass each minute. As there is a strong linear relationship between $VO_{2\,max}$ measures and endurance performance, it is often used to predict performance. Certain measures are expected by gender and training status. $VO_{2\,max}$ increases with training, and there are gender differences in measures. The gender differences are due to the physiological differences between males and females. The expected ranges of $VO_{2\,max}$ for males are 45–50 ml/kg/min for sedentary, 55–65 ml/kg/min for trained, and ≥70 ml/kg/min for elite. The expected ranges of $VO_{2\,max}$ for females are 35–40 ml/kg/min for sedentary, 45–55 ml/kg/min for trained, and ≥60 ml/kg/min for elite.

$VO_{2\,max}$ is measured during a graded exercise protocol conducted in a laboratory setting. Testing is typically conducted on either a treadmill or cycle ergometer (stationary bike). As an OCR athlete, you would conduct the graded exercise protocol on a treadmill. The graded exercise protocol starts easily, and intensity increases at regular time intervals until complete exhaustion. Most protocols consist of two- or three-minute stages. Intensity increases during the treadmill protocol by increasing both speed and grade. During the graded exercise protocol, gas exchange of O_2 and CO_2 is measured using an automated metabolic cart. This requires the participant to wear an airtight mask that allows them to breathe in room air and breathe out into a gas-mixing chamber. From the gas-mixing chamber, the air is analyzed for O_2 and CO_2.

Measurement of $VO_{2\,max}$ requires expensive specialized equipment and trained personnel to run the test and evaluate the data. Due to these facts, testing is expensive. Testing will typically run between $100 to $300 depending on the facilities, testing personnel, and other services offered. However, testing can be conducted at local performance centers and universities. The best option would be to contact the exercise physiology (kinesiology, physical education, and exercise science) department at your local university. Most researchers there are always looking for subjects and will offer low cost or free testing.

Before spending your money on $VO_{2\,max}$ testing, do your homework. I have seen a disturbing trend toward performance centers purchasing cheap metabolic carts that do not accurately measure VO_2. An accurate metabolic cart costs around $23,000, making the purchase and upkeep of the system somewhat prohibitive for many centers. Metabolic carts can be purchased for much less, but do nothing more than estimate VO_2. If the metabolic cart does not have an O_2 and CO_2 analyzer, do not waste your time, effort, or money. Prior to scheduling an appointment, ask what make and model metabolic cart will be used for testing, and do your homework. You can estimate $VO_{2\,max}$ using simple performance measures that are free and easy to accomplish. So it does not make sense to pay money to have an inaccurate machine estimate $VO_{2\,max}$.

Anaerobic and Lactate Thresholds

Threshold terminology is used a lot in sports performance, but few actually understand or know how to correctly apply the concept. The two most common terms used are "anaerobic threshold" and "lactate threshold." Anaerobic threshold is defined as the point at which metabolic processes begin a significant switch from aerobic energetics to anaerobic energetics. Lactate threshold is defined as the point at which lactate production exceeds the body's ability to remove it. Human bodies are always producing lactate, even at rest, but it is removed from the system quickly so that it does not build up. As intensity increases, lactate production increases, and there will come a point when production will exceed removal. As intensity increases, reliance on glycogen as a fuel source increases to the point that hydrogen is being produced at such a rate that it begins to build up, leading to a decrease in pH. To offset this decrease in pH, two hydrogen will bind with pyruvate to form lactic acid. This is unstable and a hydrogen is released, forming lactate.

There are two common methods for measuring lactate threshold. The first involves plotting blood lactate as intensity increases in order to determine the inflection point. The second method is referred to as onset of blood lactate accumulation and is marked at 4 millimoles per liter of blood. Using 4 millimoles per liter of blood is somewhat arbitrary and not overly accurate, however. Therefore, it is typically not used to determine threshold. To obtain lactate threshold using either method, a graded exercise protocol would be conducted where resistance is systematically increased every three minutes until exhaustion. Blood would be taken at the end of every workload and analyzed for blood lactate.

A third and less common method for determining anaerobic threshold is termed "ventilatory threshold" (VT). This is the point at which ventilation increases exponentially and is easily calculated from data collected during a $VO_{2\,max}$ test. Ventilation increases as a direct response to the increased CO_2 production that occurs due to buffering excessive hydrogen. While I have a blood lactate analyzer in my lab, I generally prefer using VT because it is accurate, easy, and I do not have to draw blood.

Regardless of the method used to determine anaerobic threshold, it will be expressed as either a percentage of max or relative to heart rate. An untrained individual can have an anaerobic threshold of about 70 percent of max, whereas an elite OCR athlete could have a threshold of around 90 percent of max. In order to use anaerobic threshold to monitor training intensity, you will need to know heart rate at threshold.

Knowing your anaerobic threshold is just as important as knowing your $VO_{2\,max}$. It can even be argued that it is more important. The higher your anaerobic threshold, the faster your race pace will be. Not only do you want to focus your training on increasing your $VO_{2\,max}$ but also on increasing your anaerobic threshold. Changes in anaerobic threshold occur quicker and have a greater impact on performance in relation to changes in $VO_{2\,max}$. Do not get me wrong, increases in both are important and should be a focus of your training plan.

TRAINING ADAPTATIONS

Adaptations to Endurance Training

Almost every adaptation that occurs due to endurance training is designed to increase the delivery of oxygen to the working muscles and increase the oxidative processes that occur within them. The entire point of your training program is to elicit these adaptations in order to improve performance. The purpose of this section is to identify the primary adaptations and explain the importance of each.

With endurance training there will be an increase in overall blood volume. Red blood cells will increase in order to boost the oxygen-carrying capacity of the blood. Plasma volume will also increase but to a greater extent. Plasma increases due to two primary reasons. The first is in response to the increased red blood cell volume. Plasma is the fluid portion of the blood responsible for the smooth transfer of the more viscous red blood cells. So if there is an increase in red blood cells, there will be a corresponding increase in plasma. Plasma volume also increases in response to the heavy sweating and plasma loss that occurs during exercise. The increased plasma volume will assist in heat dissipation and thermoregulation because there is a large increase in plasma volume in relation to the red blood cell increase; hematocrit will decrease in trained individuals.

Increased blood volume would do no good if delivery at the muscles was not also increased. In response to the greater demand, capillary density will increase at the tissue, primarily the working muscles. The increased capillary density will supply more blood to the working muscles, allowing greater gas, nutrient, and metabolic byproduct exchange.

Improved cardiac function also occurs as an adaptation to endurance training. As mentioned previously, cardiac output equals stroke volume multiplied by heart rate ($Q = SV \times HR$). With endurance training, there will be an increase in stroke volume, which affects both cardiac output and heart rate. Stroke volume increases due to three primary reasons. The first is that there will be a healthy enlargement of the left ventricle, allowing a greater volume of blood to enter. Second, the increased blood volume will result in a larger volume of blood returning to the heart and therefore greater filling. Third, the cardiac muscle will produce a more forceful contraction. Because SV has increased, there will be a corresponding decrease in HR at any submaximal intensity, because cardiac output for that given submaximal intensity has not greatly altered. This is why endurance athletes have low resting heart rates. Max heart rate does not alter with training and remains relatively constant. Due to the increase in stroke volume and no alteration in max HR, there will be an increase in cardiac output with endurance training.

Alterations to muscle fiber will also occur with endurance training. Type I muscle hypertrophy develops, leading to improved performance. Slow twitch muscle hypertrophy is often overlooked because it is not as visibly noticed in relation to the type II muscle hypertrophy that occurs due to strength and power training. Type one muscle fibers will greatly increase their oxidative capacity. Type IIa (intermediate fibers) will shift toward oxidative properties. There will also be an increase in myoglobin to increase oxygen-carrying capacity within the muscle. Mitochondria (the oxidative powerhouse of the cell) will increase, leading to an increase in oxidative processes. There will be an overall increase in all oxidative enzymes as well.

Changes to energy sources will also occur due to endurance training. There will be an increase in glycogen stores. Glycogen stores for the average individual will be around 2,000 kCals. An elite endurance athlete will store around 2,500 kCals. Lipid stores will decrease in adipose tissue and increase in muscle. This will provide greater stores in the muscles readily available for production of ATP. Lastly, you will begin to utilize fat at a higher percentage earlier during prolonged exercise in order to spare glycogen.

The last adaptation is an increase in lactate threshold, due to a decrease in lactic acid production and an increase in lactate clearance. While endurance training, especially tempo work, will increase lactate threshold, anaerobic training is key to increasing lactate threshold.

Adaptations to Anaerobic Training

Anaerobic training will result in various adaptations that will increase your anaerobic capacity, allowing you to maintain high-energy outputs for a little longer period of time. One of the main adaptations that occurs due to anaerobic training involves an increase in anaerobic threshold due to an increased buffering capacity. As mentioned previously, during high-intensity exercise, which relies on anaerobic glycolysis, hydrogen builds up in the system. This buildup of hydrogen results in a decrease in pH (increased acidity). There are two primary methods used to buffer this decrease in pH. The first is that two hydrogen will bind with pyruvate to form lactic acid, and the second is when sodium bicarbonate binds with hydrogen to form carbonic acid. When you increase your buffering capacity, you greatly increase the intensity you can compete at as well as the duration you can hold the intensity. The increase in anaerobic threshold also occurs because of an increase in glycolytic enzymes that enhances energy production through glycolysis. There is also an increase in pain tolerance in individuals who train anaerobically. With just eight weeks of high-intensity training, you can significantly increase your anaerobic threshold.

Another adaptation to anaerobic training is an increase in muscular strength. This adaptation correlates with the strongest increases in anaerobic performance. This concept has been reverse engineered by strength-and-conditioning coaches for years, with great effect. While these increases in strength from anaerobic training are great for improved performance alone, coaches have realized that implementing strength-and-power-training programs will in turn improve the athlete's anaerobic performance.

Anaerobic training will also improve motor unit recruitment and the stretch-shortening cycle, both of which will increase the muscles' ability to contract forcefully and quickly. This improvement occurs due to an increase in motor unit recruitment, an increase in the firing rate of the recruited motor units, and an improved stretch-reflex response.

Adaptations to Resistance Training

Resistance training is a vital part of your yearly training plan and will be discussed later in this book. The term "resistance training" covers muscular endurance, muscular strength, and muscular power training. When you begin a resistance training program, you will see a large increase in the first eight weeks of training. Keep in mind that eight weeks is an average number that assumes you have not been previously active in resistance training. When someone new to resistance training begins a program, they will see somewhat steady gains for about the first eight weeks and then level off. This is because the first eight weeks of training result in neuromuscular adaptations that improve performance without a correlating increase in muscle fiber size (hypertrophy). These neuromuscular adaptations consist of increased motor unit recruitment, increased synchronization of motor unit and muscle activation, and a reduction in the golgi tendon organ (the sensory organ that limits force development as a protective mechanism) threshold. It is important to understand this concept so that you do not become frustrated when your gains level off and then proceed at a much slower pace. This phenomenon is normal and to be expected.

After the first eight weeks of resistance training, you will begin to see increases in muscle fiber diameter (hypertrophy). To understand hypertrophy, it is important to first have an understanding of basic muscle structure. A muscle is made up of fasciculi bound together by connective tissue. Each individual fasciculus is made up of a bundle of muscle fiber, and each muscle fiber is made up of a bundle of myofibril. Within the myofibril you have actin and myosin, which work together to cause a contraction of the muscle. Hypertrophy occurs due to an increase in the number of actin and myosin within each myofibril and an increase in the number of myofibril within each muscle fiber. To date, there is no strong evidence to support an increase in the number of muscle fibers within a muscle (hyperplasia) in humans.

PSYCHOLOGICAL TRAINING

We focus so much on the physiological and biomechanical principles of sport and often overlook the psychological factors of sport performance. Your psychological state can directly impact your physiological performance on many levels. For example, your heart rate will increase in anticipation of a workout or competition without any increase in physical demand. The greater the anxiety, the higher your heart rate will be prior to participation. There is nothing wrong with an anticipatory increase in heart rate, and as a matter of fact, starting your warm-up with a higher heart rate is beneficial. This section is not designed to give you an in-depth knowledge of sport psychology, but instead will hit on some key factors that will help with your performance.

Anxiety

Anxiety is a feeling of apprehension, nervousness, or fear that is in response to an event. While anxiety is a psychological construct, there is a corresponding physiological response. Anxiety results in an increased activity of the sympathetic nervous system, leading to an increase in cardiac output, redirection of blood flow, tightening of muscles, and gastrointestinal distress. It is quite common to feel anxious about an upcoming competition or event, and everyone experiences anxiety prior to a race.

Being anxious is not entirely a bad thing as it triggers your fight or flight response and prepares your body for the competition. However, it is not good to be overly anxious. Focusing on your anxiety prevents you from focusing on the competition at hand and can lead to negative physiological responses (tight muscles, gastrointestinal distress, etc.).

Attention and Focus

When training for and competing in OCR, it is important to focus on the trail so that you can pick the ideal path along the trail and respond to any obstacles. Your body will go in the direction of your focus. If you are running at the edge of a ditch and your focus is on the ditch and not the trail, you will start moving toward the ditch. Instead, focus your attention on where you want to go and not where you do not wish to go. When attacking obstacles, it is important to focus your attention on the next hand or foot placement in order to securely place your hold. "Selective attention" is the term used to describe an athlete's focus on performance-relative cues while ignoring all nonessential cues. It is important to block out all the commotion going on around you and focus on the trail and obstacles in front of you.

Visualization

If you can visualize a movement or a sequence of movements, it will greatly increase your ability to perform those movements. This theory holds true for anything from climbing a rope to throwing the javelin. Visualizing the movement in your head as you produce the movement allows you to better conduct the movement. In order to effectively use visualization, it is vital that you know and understand the appropriate sequencing of the techniques.

The ability to correctly use visualization is a learned process and takes time to master. Video recordings of performance can help the athlete with visualization. Often, with beginners, it is hard to visualize proper technique. For example, a coach will explain to an athlete that he or she is conducting the technique incorrectly and the athlete does not understand because he or she feels it in fact is being done correctly. When the coach shows the athlete the video and details what is being done incorrectly, the athlete can now better visualize what to change as well as the correct technique.

Desensitization

Desensitization is the process by which you work to reduce the impact of a stimulus. It is a normal human reaction to feel fear when climbing or traversing heights. Although that is a normal reaction, it is counterproductive to effectively competing in obstacle course racing. With time and training you will become desensitized to these factors and respond more appropriately. However, this does not mean that you should be fearless. A little fear is a good thing.

To work on the desensitization process, simply get accustomed to those factors of OCR that scare you. For example, if you are afraid of heights, then slowly work higher and higher until you are completely comfortable. If you are afraid of the water obstacles, work on becoming more comfortable in the water. The more time you spend in the water, the more confident you will become.

Motivation

Motivation is the force that drives the way you respond to situations. Motivation is not always simple and straightforward. Often motivation is multifaceted, complicated, and not always clear. Everyone reading this book will have different motivations for becoming involved in obstacle course racing. Some will become involved for the competition, others will use it as a tool to get in shape, and still others simply for the self-challenge. Most often, though, there is more than one factor that motivates someone to get involved. Taking the time to sit down and understand your motivation to train will allow you to better focus on your training plan and long-term goals.

Motivation can either be intrinsic (from within) or extrinsic (from outside sources). Intrinsic motivation will have the largest impact on your performance in the long run as the focus comes from your own desires. Intrinsic motivation is driven by your desire to excel, curiosity, love of the sport, desire to learn, desire to be challenged, etc. As your desires are self-motivated, it is less likely that you will experience burnout or frequent changes in attitude toward training and competing. Intrinsic motivation leads to greater learning, greater focus, greater self-confidence, and greater satisfaction.

Extrinsic motivation can be either beneficial or harmful to performance. Examples of extrinsic motivation are monetary reward, trophies, external praise or lack thereof (from a coach, parents, friends, etc.), contract or scholarship, etc. The problem with extrinsic motivation is that it is completely out of the athlete's control, and there is a danger that the athlete will focus their self-worth on these extrinsic factors. Extrinsic motivators can also lead to anxiety. Extrinsic motivators work best when the athlete has strong intrinsic motivation and the extrinsic motivation is not overemphasized. Also, those who focus solely on extrinsic motivators will burn out easier and will not develop as quickly.

Setting Goals

When developing a program, it is important to establish long- and short-term goals in order to develop a long-range training plan. When working with a new athlete, I first want to know their long-term goals. This allows me to determine their overall motivation for training and to build a successful program for them to reach those goals. It is difficult to develop a plan without knowing where you want to go.

Goals should be challenging, while remaining realistic and attainable. It is okay to set a high goal, such as becoming a professional racer. However, it is not realistic to set the goal for your first year of training. It is always a good idea to talk over your goals with your coach so that you can get them set and develop a plan. In order to set your goals, ask yourself the following questions:

- Overall, what do I want to accomplish?
  - fitness
  - competition
  - being outdoors
  - combination of any of the three
- What is my current fitness level?
- What is my current skill level?
- How much time can I dedicate to training?
- What are my logistical challenges?

These are some of the basic questions you can use to help determine your goals. It is important to think about each question and answer each as honestly as possible.

As mentioned, when setting goals, it is important to set both short- and long-term goals. Look at it like a ladder. If you only had the bottom and top rungs of the ladder, it would be virtually useless, and you would be unable to climb to the top (your ultimate goal). Adding rungs (short-term goals) to the ladder between the bottom and the top will allow you to climb easily and ultimately reach your goal. The journey to reach your ultimate goal can be difficult, long, and at times discouraging. Short-term goals give you something to strive for along the way.

After determining your long-term and short-term goals, write them down so that you will have them for future reference. The act of writing down your goals makes it much more likely that you will stick to those goals. Place your goals where you can see them daily so that they will provide motivation along your journey.

Do Not Make Comparisons

One of the worst mistakes OCR athletes will make is to compare their progression with the performance level of other racers. This is doubly true when a beginner attempts to compare their current level to an elite-level racer. It is important to remember that the elite racer started where you currently stand and progressed to an elite level through hard training and dedication. Do not focus on whether you are better than someone else. Instead, focus on whether you are better today than you were yesterday. If the answer is yes, then you are going in the right direction. If the answer is no, then you need to evaluate your motivation, consistency, and training plan to determine why you are not progressing, and then make appropriate changes.

This concept does not mean that you should not realistically determine where your performance level is in relation to others if you plan to compete. Never compete before you are ready as it may lead to disappointment if your performance level is not where it needs to be.

3

AREAS OF TRAINING

This chapter will cover the various areas of training you should focus on in order to improve your obstacle course racing. While cardiorespiratory endurance is a primary component of OCR, there are other areas you should focus on in order to optimally complete obstacles. Some obstacles will require muscular endurance, while others will require strength or power.

AEROBIC TRAINING

Aerobic training is designed to improve your cardiorespiratory endurance, which is a primary component of obstacle course racing; therefore, a large portion of your training will be in this area. As mentioned previously, determining training intensity is important if you want to improve your performance. The majority of your training will be conducted below anaerobic threshold, with a small portion at or above threshold. The following methods can be used to control training intensity.

Determining Intensity Using Speed or Pace

Speed and pace are often used to regulate intensity when running. Speed is measured in miles per hour, and pace is measured in minutes per mile. For example, if you run a 5k (3.1 miles) in 21 minutes, then your pace would be 6:46 per mile and your speed would be 8.85 mph. A modern GPS can provide both your pace and speed. As obstacle course racing is conducted on trails, using speed or pace to determine intensity could be misleading, however, as it is easier to maintain an overall faster speed on a flat, rolling course than on a course that requires a lot of climbing. This factor makes it impossible to compare intensities between two different trails when using pace or speed. However, you can compare speeds between different runs on the same trail.

While using speed has its drawbacks, it is still an easy and practical tool. But do not fall into the trap of trying to obtain a personal best every time you run. You should stick with the specific goal of that training session and make adjustments only based on the environmental conditions. Keep in mind that you should not compare average speeds from one course with another.

Time can be used as a marker set for improved performance. To do this, run the course at race pace and then repeat the course on a separate day in similar environmental conditions. If times are faster, then you know the program is working. However, if times have declined or have not improved, look at your training and recovery program to determine if changes need to be made. There will be bad days when your performance is not good, but a single bad day does not mean your program is not working. If you have a bad marker set, take a few days to recover, and then try the marker set again. If you still have a lower performance, then reevaluate your training program.

Marker sets should be performed periodically and not every time you are on the trail. Treat a marker set as a race. Make sure that you are well recovered, well hydrated, well fueled, and well rested prior to any marker set. Your goal is to measure improvements in performance and not how tired you are from your interval training the previous day or the fact that you only got three hours of sleep the night prior.

Determining Intensity by Using Heart Rate

Using heart rate to determine intensity may seem a little daunting. However, it is a very easy method to implement into your training and is a good tool for setting levels of intensity. Heart rate shares a linear relationship with intensity from rest to maximal effort, meaning that as intensity increases, so too does heart rate in equal measure.

Recently, though, there has been a trend toward not relying on heart rate for determining intensity levels, due to the day-to-day variability in heart rate. While it is true that heart rate varies from day to day, it does not invalidate heart rate as a useful tool. Being aware of normal heart rate variability allows you to better understand heart rate and better implement heart rate monitoring into your training program.

Hydration levels and recovery strongly impact heart rate. As you become dehydrated, blood plasma volume decreases, which in turn leads to a decrease in stroke volume (volume of blood ejected from the heart with each beat). A decrease in stroke volume results in an increase in heart rate at any resting or submaximal (also known as submax) intensity level. Endurance athletes who are training in the summer have a tendency to stay chronically dehydrated. On long hot rides, heart rate can gradually increase due to dehydration.

Heart rate will also remain elevated during recovery from training due to replenishing energy systems, cooling the body, and anabolic (tissue-building) processes. During easy days, heart rate returns to resting levels fairly quickly. However, after a hard day of training, resting and submax heart rates can remain elevated for a period of time.

One last factor to keep in mind is cardiovascular drift, which is an increase in heart rate without an increase in intensity during prolonged steady exercise, particularly in a hot environment. Cardiovascular drift is typically a result of dehydration. During prolonged exercise, plasma volume decreases due to sweating, which leads to a decrease in blood volume, resulting in a decrease in blood return to the heart and a subsequent decrease in stroke volume. In order to dissipate heat from the body's core, more blood will be sent to the skin for cooling, which also decreases venous return and stroke volume. Cardiac output (volume of blood ejected from the heart each minute) is the product of heart rate and stroke volume. Because cardiac output must be maintained in order to sustain a specific intensity, heart rate must increase to compensate for the decrease in stroke volume. Do not be surprised if your heart rate begins to creep up on a long run, especially if it is hot outside.

A heart rate monitor is the best method for measuring heart rate, because it detects the electrical impulse of the heart contractions. You can also count pulse rate at either the carotid artery (located at the neck) or the radial artery (located at the wrist). However, this method is not as accurate when compared to using a heart rate monitor. When purchasing a monitor, look for one with a chest transmitter as they are the most accurate.

To use heart rate as a training tool, you need an anchor point. The most common anchor point used is heart rate max. Heart rate max is the highest heart rate measured at maximal intensity. In order to determine your max heart rate, either conduct a $VO_{2\,max}$ test or perform hill repeats at maximal effort. $VO_{2\,max}$ testing requires specialized equipment and provides a greater amount of information than performing hill repeats.

But you do not need a laboratory or sophisticated equipment to determine max heart rate. You can simply perform hill repeats at maximal intensity. Find a hill that is about a quarter to half a mile long. Warm up for about 15 to 30 minutes, and then run the hill as fast as possible. If you are not completely exhausted at the top of the climb, you did not run hard enough. The idea here is to achieve your max heart rate. Repeat the climb two to four times and record the highest heart rate achieved. Upon completion, cool down by running easily for 10 to 15 minutes.

The problem with using intervals to determine max heart rate is that it requires you to repeatedly engage in maximal effort bouts. This is not typically recommended for beginners; you may want to consider estimating max heart rate instead. There are various formulas that will help you make a close estimate. These formulas are not overly accurate but will provide a ballpark anchor point that will be relatively accurate for most individuals. Once you establish a good training plan and fitness level, I recommend ditching the estimated max HR and conducting hill repeats or a $VO_{2\,max}$ test in order to determine your true max heart rate.

Example Formula
$220 - age = HR_{max}$
Example: $220 - 41$ years of age = 179 beats per minute (bpm)
$210 - (age \times .5) - (body\ weight\ in\ pounds \times .05) + correction\ factor = HR_{max}$
Correction factor = + 4 for males and + 0 for females
$210 - (41 \times .5) - (180 \times .05) + 4 = 184.5$ bpm

Now that you have established max heart rate, you will next need to determine intensity based on heart rate. Training zone heart rates will set the parameters of your training session for that day by providing an upper and lower heart rate limit. This is where a training zone alarm on your heart rate monitor comes into play. It will allow you to train without constantly checking your monitor to determine if you are in or out of your training zone. Here are four basic heart rate training zones:

Zone 1—Active Recovery

- 50 to 65 percent of max heart rate.
- Beginners will typically stay closer to 50 percent.
- Training below 70 percent ensures that it is an active recovery day.

Zone 2—Aerobic

- 70 to 80 percent of max heart rate.
- For beginners, 80 percent may be too high and you may want to consider staying closer to 70 percent.
- This is where the majority of your training will occur.

Zone 3—Threshold

- 80 to 90 percent of max heart rate.
- This will be your race pace or tempo training.

Zone 4—Interval

- 90 to 100 percent of max heart rate.
- This will be your high-intensity training above threshold.

You can also set heart rate training zones using heart rate at anaerobic threshold. If you know the heart rate that corresponds to your current anaerobic threshold, you can set training zones based on that anchor point. Anaerobic threshold will change with training, and the better race shape you are in, the higher your anaerobic threshold will be. The common four zones when using threshold heart rate are:

Zone 1—Active Recovery	25 percent or more below threshold heart rate
Zone 2—Aerobic	25 to 10 percent below threshold heart rate
Zone 3—Threshold	± 10 percent of threshold heart rate
Zone 4—Interval	> 110 percent of heart rate threshold

The reason that an upper and lower heart rate is given with each training zone is due to day-to-day heart rate variability, which makes it somewhat impossible to stay at a single fixed heart rate for each given zone. The majority of your endurance training will focus on heart rate training zones one and two. Naturally, if you are running up a steep hill you may have to go out of your zone in order to run the hill. However, it's best if you can slow down and take the hill easier to stay within or closer to your zone.

Heart rate training in zone three (race pace) becomes a little more complicated. As an obstacle course racer, it is important to learn to pace yourself on feel and known distance in a race situation. Obstacle course racing is a self-paced event, and you will develop pacing strategies. Use of a heart rate monitor to control intensity during a race may limit your race performance. Instead, learn to pace based on how you feel at race pace. You may still want to wear a heart rate monitor during the race in order to evaluate performance afterward.

When coaching, I was not concerned about heart rate during interval training and typically used time to run a fixed distance for intervals. Intervals are conducted at high intensities, and heart rate can even continue to climb briefly after a high-intensity interval.

Determining Intensity by Feel

Determining intensity based on feel is a valuable tool that is often applied incorrectly or overlooked altogether. Endurance athletes who have been racing for a while are able to pace correctly for different training zones based on known distance and how they feel (peripheral feedback). Beginners typically have a difficult time correctly gauging intensity, especially during a race. They may go out too fast, experience fatigue, and then slow down, leading to a poor performance time. Using an even-paced race strategy is ideal for endurance sports. During an obstacle course race, effort will alter greatly with terrain. However, you can keep an even pacing strategy by basing it on how you feel.

There are a couple simple methods that help you to control intensity through feel, the first of which is the talk test, which is extremely simple to use and, yet, very effective. The talk test allows you to determine if you are below, at, or above threshold. If you are training below threshold, you should be able to hold a decent conversation. The closer you get to threshold, the harder it will be to hold a conversation. At threshold you should only be able to get out a short sentence at most. Above threshold you may get out one or two words at most.

The next method, a bit more complicated, uses a rating of perceived exertion (RPE) scale to determine intensity (numbered scale indicating level of fatigue). You can use the Borg scale, one of the most common RPE scales used in exercise science, which runs from a rating of 6 (no exertion) to 20 (maximal exertion), to correlate to an average resting heart rate of 60 bpm and max heart rate of 200 bpm. Or, use the OMNI scale (rating of 0 [extremely easy] to 10 [extremely hard]), which has become the preferred RPE scale because it is more logical in nature.

Prior to using an RPE scale to determine training intensity, and accurately correlate an RPE number to how you feel, it is important to first anchor it during a graded exercise protocol. A graded exercise protocol starts off at an easy level and increases intensity every two to three minutes (depending on the protocol). During the graded exercise protocol, you will establish an RPE every minute by determining how you feel at that point. This allows you to anchor all numbers from first to last.

As you become more experienced, you will not need the talk test or an RPE scale and will be able to control your race pace based on the known distance and how you feel during the race. You will be able to find that sweet spot that maximizes your performance and gives you the power you need as you cross the finish line.

ANAEROBIC TRAINING

Anaerobic training is the high-intensity training that will be conducted above threshold in order to improve your anaerobic capacity. When looking at OCR from a metabolic perspective, it is an aerobic event with many anaerobic bouts throughout the race, so interval training is the best method for increasing your anaerobic abilities.

There are multiple ways to conduct interval training, and I will discuss a few of those methods. To begin, most endurance athletes conduct interval training incorrectly. They go out as hard as they can each interval with their overall output decreasing and time per interval increasing with every subsequent interval. This is called overreaching interval training, and it has a place within a well-designed program. However, the mistake most athletes make is that they conduct overreaching intervals every time they conduct intervals. The majority of your interval training should be conducted so that the last interval is at the same pace as the first interval, but you can barely hold the prescribed pace during the last interval. If you can barely hold the prescribed pace during the first interval, then your pace will continuously drop throughout the remaining intervals. The first through last intervals should be conducted at a level that is challenging, yet allows you to maintain the assigned pace for every interval.

You can conduct either long or short intervals. Short intervals could be anywhere from 100 to 400m. This type of interval really pushes an athlete's anaerobic abilities. Set shorter intervals so that your pace is about 60 to 90 seconds faster than your 5k race pace. For example, if you run a 21-minute 5k, then your pace is 6:46 per mile. If you subtract 90 seconds, you end up with a 5:16 per mile pace. Next, divide that time by 4 and you'll have a 1:19 pace for a 400m interval. This will give you a starting point. Keep in mind that while the intervals should be challenging, you should be able to complete the first and last intervals at the same pace. If you cannot, then slow your intervals down. If the workout was too easy, just speed the intervals up during your next session.

You can also do longer interval sessions (800 to 1,600 meters) to increase your threshold for race pace. For longer intervals, drop 10 to 30 seconds off your race pace. Using the same example from above, if you run a 21-minute 5k, then your pace is 6:46 per mile. If you subtract 30 seconds you end up with a 6:16 per mile pace. Next, divide that time by 2 and you'll have a 3:08 pace for an 800m interval. Again, you will need to adjust pace so that you complete your intervals at the correct intensity.

A rest period between intervals is another key concept to consider when conducting interval training. You must make sure that energy systems and neuromuscular fatigue are addressed between bouts. However, currently there is no concrete evidence to state what the exact work-to-rest ratio should be at different interval time lengths. The typical recommendation is that the work-to-rest ratio for intervals that are 60 to 120 seconds in length should be approximately 1:3, and for intervals that are about 3 to 5 minutes, the work-to-rest ratio should be 1:1. So, if you are conducting a 60-second interval (work), then your recovery should be 180 seconds (rest). If you are conducting 5-minute intervals (work), then your recovery should be 5 minutes (rest). The rest interval can either be conducted actively (very easy running/walking) or passively (no running/walking). Either will work, but I tend to recommend active recovery during long sessions. Keep in mind that active here actually means that you are running/walking very easily and slowly for recovery.

You can also conduct fartlek sessions where the intervals are not timed specifically and instead you pick up the pace at random intervals and recover in between. Typically, I recommend that you feel well recovered, but not necessarily completely recovered, between intervals. This can be something fun that you do with your friends. Assign everyone a number, one through however many are running with you, and the intervals start in numerical order. Line up by number and start down the trail. When the first runner decides to start the interval, they quickly pick up speed without a word, and everyone else attempts to keep up. During the recovery phase, the first runner goes to the back of the line and then runner two will decide when to pick up the pace again. Keep repeating this process throughout the run. Make sure that the slowest runner is recovered before starting the next acceleration. Remember, not everyone will be at the same fitness level and the goal is to have fun and not to crush each other.

Overreaching intervals can be used periodically to maximize stress on the physiological systems of your body. Unlike normal interval training, overreaching intervals will have continuously slower intervals as the training session progresses. Each interval is conducted as fast as you can run, which will result in slower intervals as you fatigue with each subsequent interval. Overreaching intervals should be used sparingly as they place high stress on the body.

RESISTANCE TRAINING

Obstacle course racing requires a lot of muscular endurance and strength in order to successfully navigate the obstacles. This section will start by discussing training for the common obstacles you will encounter during an obstacle course race. It would be impractical to include every possible obstacle; therefore, I will focus only on the most common. As you read, keep in mind that this section will discuss strength and conditioning for various obstacles and the actual skill for traversing individual obstacles will be covered later in this book.

There are a few key concepts to keep in mind as you read through this section. One of the first is that you must be able to manage your body weight with your upper body, lower body, and a combination of both under varying circumstances. Another is that both training for the specific obstacles and working the primary muscles involved in those obstacles are very important as both are key components for improvement. Lastly, most obstacles you will encounter require a pulling movement, which can result in muscular imbalances. Therefore, it is important to include muscles involved in pushing in your workout program in order to maintain that balance. Muscular imbalances often result in overuse injuries.

Obstacles

In this section, the obstacles discussed will be divided into four common categories. The training advice here will provide you sport-specific training for competing in obstacle course racing. The individual obstacles will not be discussed in detail, however, and the skills required to effectively complete individual obstacles will be discussed in chapter 7.

Overhead

One of the most common categories of obstacles that you will be challenged with on a racing course is the overhead obstacle. Some of the most common overhead obstacles are the monkey bars, rings, floating bars, dials, and ropes. Often there will be a combination of more than one type in a single obstacle.

These types of obstacles require that you traverse an area while hanging by your hands from the obstacle, without the use of your feet and without touching the ground. Overhead obstacles require the use of muscles that cause finger and wrist flexion (flexor digitorum superficialis, flexor digitorum profundus, flexor carpi radialis, palmaris, longus, etc.), and therefore grip strength is vitally important. Overhead obstacles also use muscles that are used in pull-ups (latissimus dorsi, rhomboids, teres major, biceps brachii, and brachioradialis), which makes the pull-up an ideal exercise for improving performance in this area.

Training for overhead obstacles is an excellent example of the principle of specificity: train the way you want your body to adapt. If you want to do well during overhead obstacles, you need to train for them, while adding resistance movements that mimic the movement that occurs during an obstacle. Pull-ups, lat pull-downs, and rowing are excellent examples of resistance movements that will help you focus on improving performance with overhead obstacles.

Climbing

Climbing obstacles are another common obstacle you will encounter while racing. When comparing climbing obstacles to overhead obstacles, you will find that the upper body movements are very similar and require the same muscles; however, the difference is that you can use your feet to help you with the climb. Some of the common climbing obstacles are the rope climb, cargo net climb, log climb, and handhold wall climbs. While each scenario is unique, they have basic movements in common.

The lower body will provide upward momentum as the legs extend to move upward against gravity. The primary lower body muscles involved in most climbing events are the quadricep muscles, the hamstring muscles, the gluteus muscles, and the triceps surae. These muscles are commonly used during exercise movements such as squats and plyometric jumping.

Weighted Carry

Another common obstacle used in OCR is the weighted carry. This is an event in which an object is picked up and carried a specified distance. Of course, the objects are never light. One example is the bucket carry. When conducting the bucket carry, you must maintain an isometric contraction with the trapezius, levator scapula, rhomboids, erector spinae muscles, abdominal muscles, biceps brachii, and flexor muscles of the fingers and wrists. The muscles of the lower body (gluteus muscles, hamstrings, quadriceps, and triceps surae) will contract dynamically as you move.

Carrying weighted objects should be worked into your training program to prepare you for this event. You can accomplish this by purchasing a 5-gallon bucket from your local hardware store and filling it to the desired weight. Placing a lid on the bucket will prevent the contents from spilling out as you train. For sandbag carries, buy a bag of sand and then wrap it in heavy plastic bags at the desired weight to prevent losing any of the sand while you train. When conducting the weighted carry during training, it is important that you do not overload the weight. Start off with a light weight and then work your way up. When carrying an object, keep the weight as close to your center of gravity as possible. The farther away it is from your center of gravity, the less stable you become, which will require more effort on your part. Keep strong posture throughout the carry. If you feel your posture giving, then it is time to stop and recover before your next set or stop and lower the weight for the next set.

One of the best supplemental exercises that will help you with the weighted carry is the deadlift. The deadlift utilizes all the same muscles as the weighted carry and will greatly improve your performance. Squats and shrugs are two more exercises that will help you improve your performance in this event. These exercises will be described later in this chapter.

Low Crawl

Most obstacle course races will have some form of the low crawl. The most common is the barbed-wire low crawl. Training for low crawl obstacles is often overlooked, but you can fatigue quickly in a race if you do not train properly. Muscles involved with the low crawl are the quadriceps, hamstrings, triceps surae, hip flexors, latissimus dorsi, pectoralis major, deltoids, triceps, and core. There are various muscular endurance exercises that you can use to improve your performance during low crawl obstacles. Some of the most common (army low crawl, alligator crawl, and bear crawl) will be discussed later in this chapter.

Resistance Training Exercises

When weight lifting for resistance training, each lift requires specific techniques, but there are general guidelines that go with all lifts:

- Maintain proper technique throughout the movements. Don't try to use momentum to get through a lift when the resistance is too heavy. If the resistance is heavy enough to require you to alter proper form, you should decrease the weight to maintain form.

- Movements should be conducted in a controlled manner and at a constant speed. The speed should not be explosive and fast, nor should it be super slow.
- Correctly grip the bar at all times in order to prevent the bar from rolling out of your hands.
- Do not attempt to lift weights that are too heavy for your current fitness level. This is a common source of injury. Remember to let your ego go. It does not matter how much you are lifting as you are not training to be a power lifter; you are training to be the best obstacle racer you can become.
- Work large muscle groups before working small muscle groups. If you work the small muscle groups first, they will become too fatigued to allow you to adequately work the large muscle groups. For example, if you work the triceps brachii first and then work the pectoralis major, the triceps will be too fatigued and give out prior to the pectoralis major fatiguing. Instead, work the pectoralis major first and then the triceps.
- Never hold your breath. Inhale during the eccentric load and exhale during the concentric load. Holding your breath during a lift will result in a larger spike in blood pressure than normal (blood pressure always spikes during lifting), which will cause a large decrease in blood pressure when the lift stops, resulting in dizziness.
- For safety always use a spotter with free weights.
- Use collars on the barbells in order to keep the weight from shifting on the bar. It only takes a slight shift in the bar to cause a weight to slide, which results in a catastrophic event as the plates start sliding off the bar.

Resistance training should be conducted two to three days per week—typically Monday, Wednesday, and Friday. Not all three of those days have to be in the weight room lifting weights. You can work in plyometrics or sports-specific resistance training during one of those sessions. There will be phases of training when you focus on increasing muscular strength and lift, and there will be phases when you are focusing on sport-specific obstacle training only.

The next step is to determine your sets and repetitions. Sets are the number of times you perform the exercise, and repetition is the number of times you lift or perform the movement per set. Since you want to get in and out, I typically recommend two sets for the majority of exercises in the program.

I recommend 8 to 15 repetitions when lifting weights. When conducting body management exercises (muscular endurance: push-ups, crunches, etc.), the goal is muscular endurance, and therefore do not limit yourself to 8 to 15 repetitions. Instead, do as many as you can with the goal of conducting at least one more repetition each training session. For example, if you conducted 16 pull-ups on your first set on Monday, then your goal should be at least 17 reps on the first set during your workout on Wednesday.

Determine weight based on desired repetitions. For example, if you are conducting two sets with goal repetitions of 8 to 15, you would set the weight so that volitional exhaustion occurs between 8 and 15 reps for both sets. This may take you a couple of workouts to determine. If you are able to conduct more than 15 repetitions, then increase the weight. If you cannot conduct at least 8 repetitions, then decrease the weight.

The next step is to choose the resistance exercises. Below are examples of exercises that you can implement into your resistance training program. Research has shown that improvements occur with lifting, plyometrics, body management exercises, and sports-specific exercises. I typically use a mixture of all of them. These are just a few exercise examples to get you started. If you are serious about your performance, consider hiring a strength-and-conditioning coach.

Work your entire body, including the upper body, lower body, and core; avoid focusing on one area and ignoring others. The lifts and exercises listed below supply a sufficient program to cover all the major muscle groups that are important for obstacle course racing. You do not have to use all the resistance exercises listed below. Choose the ones that work best with your desired outcome. You can replace these lifts with others that work the same muscles, or focus more on a specific area by adding more lifts into your program. If you are not familiar with the muscles involved with each specific lift, then I strongly recommend purchasing a book that shows the specific muscles used in each movement.

Start with large muscle groups and then follow up with small muscles. For example, work the bench press prior to working triceps exercises. If you fatigue the triceps by conducting triceps extension prior to doing bench, then you will not be able to adequately work the pectoralis major due to triceps fatigue.

Resistance Training Exercises

Bench Press

The pectoralis major, anterior deltoids, and triceps brachii are the primary muscles used in the bench press (see fig. 3.1). Other muscles used in this lift are

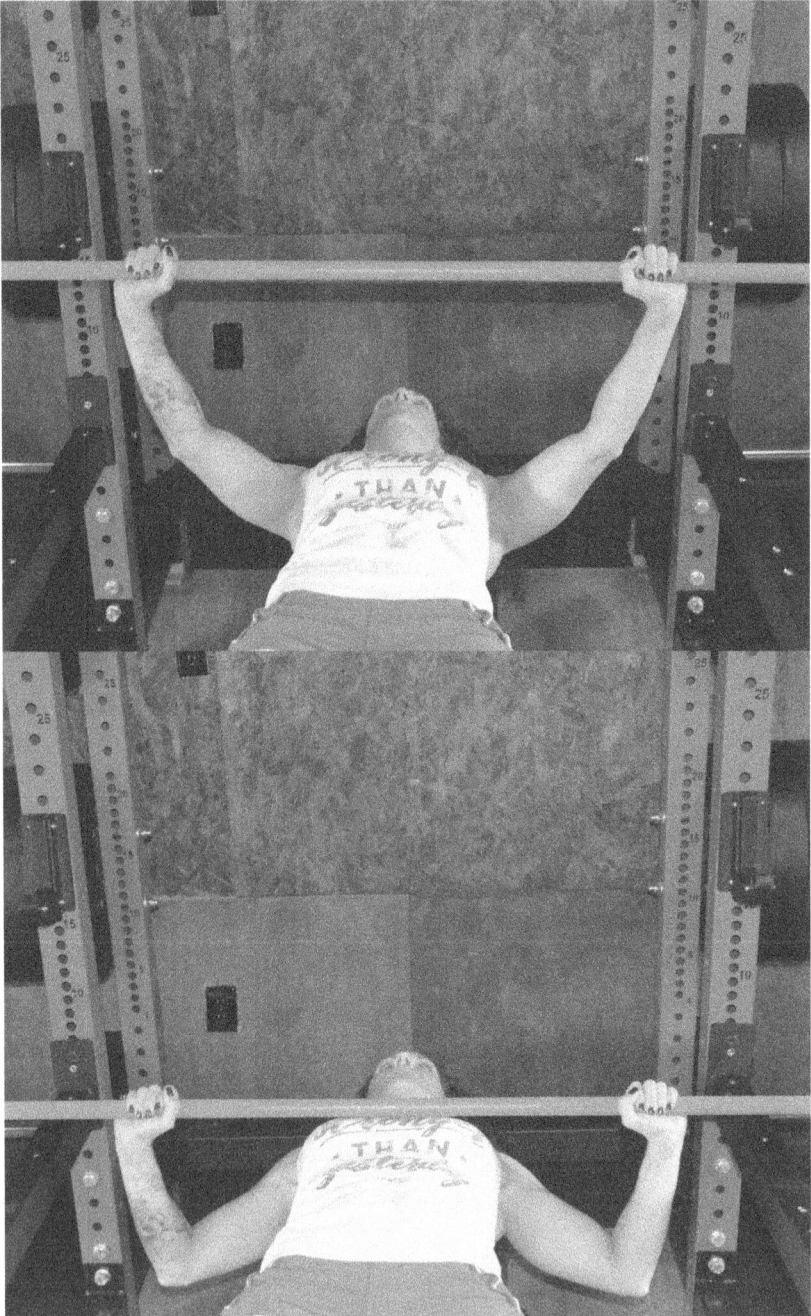

Figure 3.1.   Bench press. *Will and Renee Peveler.*

the serratus anterior and coracobrachialis. In order to conduct the bench press, lie flat on your back with both feet planted on the floor. Place your hands on the bar about shoulder-width apart with the palms facing away and fingers and thumbs wrapped around the bar. Begin by lowering the weight until it is about 1 inch from your chest. Do not bounce the weight off your chest. From the lowered position, push the weight back up to the start position.

Lat Pull-Down

The lat pull-down is designed to work the latissimus dorsi, teres major, and biceps brachii, as shown in fig. 3.2. Adjust the lat pull-down machine per the manufacturer's instruction. Grab the bar just wider than shoulder width so that your palms are facing away from you. Pull the bar down in front of your head, and then return to the start position.

Seated Row

The latissimus dorsi, trapezius, rhomboids (major and minor), teres major, posterior deltoids, and biceps brachii are worked during the seated row (see fig. 3.3). Adjust the machine per the manufacturer's instructions. Begin by bringing the bar/handles to your chest and then returning to the start position. Maintain proper back posture throughout the movement.

Overhead Press

The overhead press (see fig. 3.4) can be conducted either seated or standing. The deltoid, pectoralis major (clavicular head only), and triceps are the primary muscles used during this exercise. When conducted on a machine, follow the manufacturer's instructions. The overhead press can also be conducted using dumbbells. Grab the dumbbells in an overhand grip and place them a little higher than shoulder level with the back of the hand facing you. This is the start position. Press up over the head and then return to the start position. Overhead press can also be conducted with a barbell, but I recommend beginners stick with dumbbells. Dumbbells allow more natural joint movement throughout the lift.

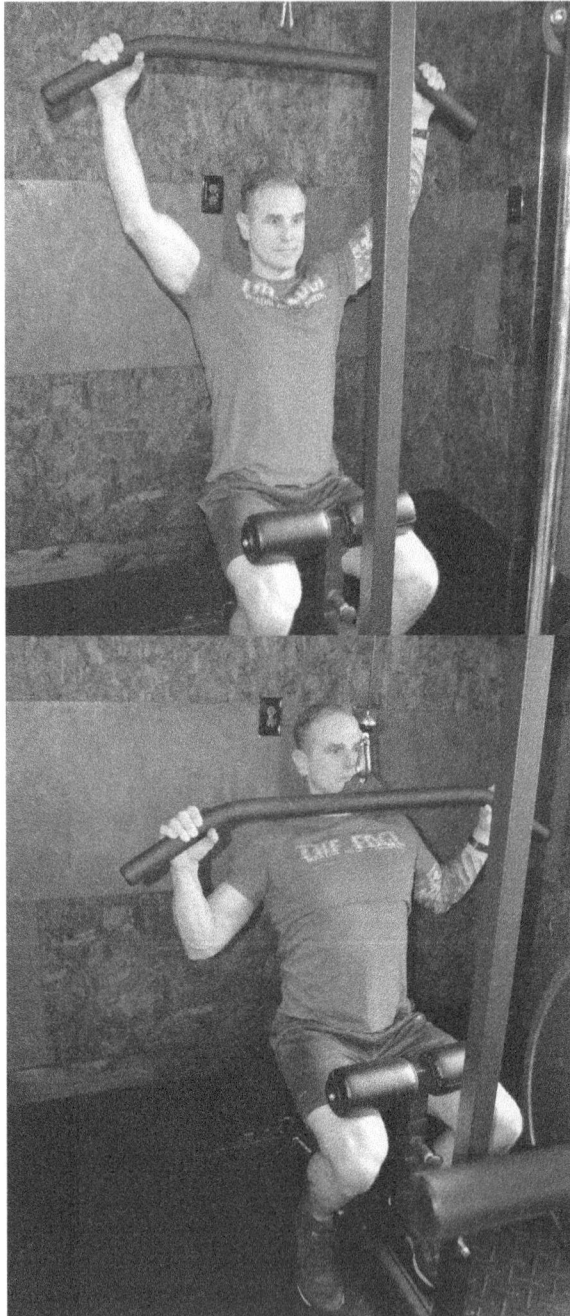

Figure 3.2.   Lat pull-down. *Will and Renee Peveler.*

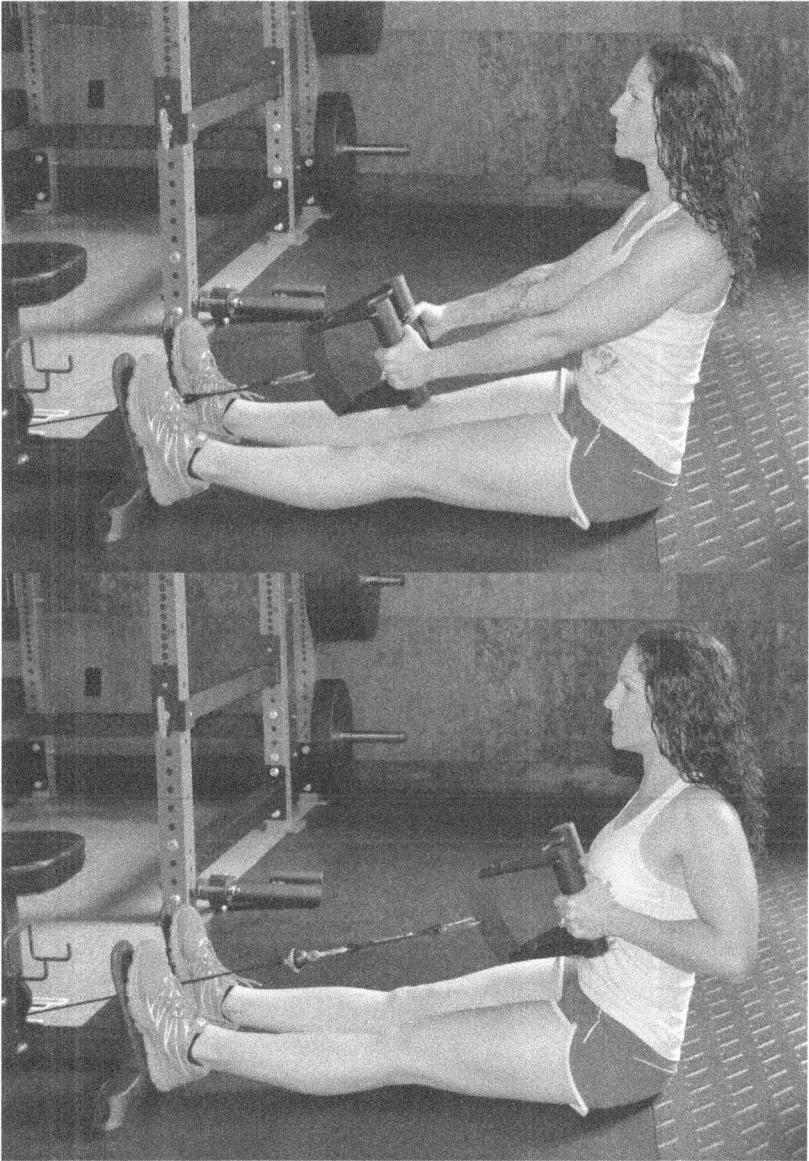

Figure 3.3.   Seated row. *Will and Renee Peveler*.

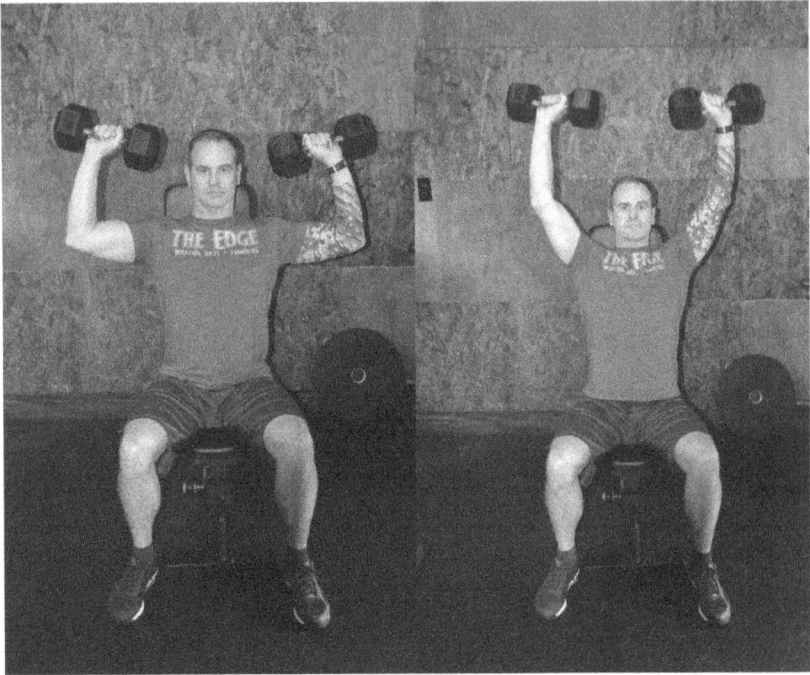

Figure 3.4. Overhead press. *Will and Renee Peveler.*

Squats

The primary muscles used during the squat are the quadriceps, hamstrings, and gluteus maximus (see fig. 3.5). The first step in conducting the squat is to adjust the squat rack height so that you can easily take the bar off and put it back when the set is complete. When conducting the squat, center the bar across the back and shoulders and grab the bar with both hands. Choose a hand position that provides both comfort and control of the bar. Lift the bar off the rack and back up into position, making sure to stay over the safety bars. Place your feet shoulder-width apart. During the lowering phase, do not allow your knees to move forward beyond your feet. Lower into the squatted position until your thighs are parallel to the floor. Next push up with the legs, returning to the standing position. When pushing up, drive through your heels, keeping the weight centered. When you reach the top of the lift, do not lock your knees. In order to maintain proper posture, make sure that you do not look down with your head as it will shift your center of gravity forward. Keep your head looking forward or slightly up, and drive with your heels.

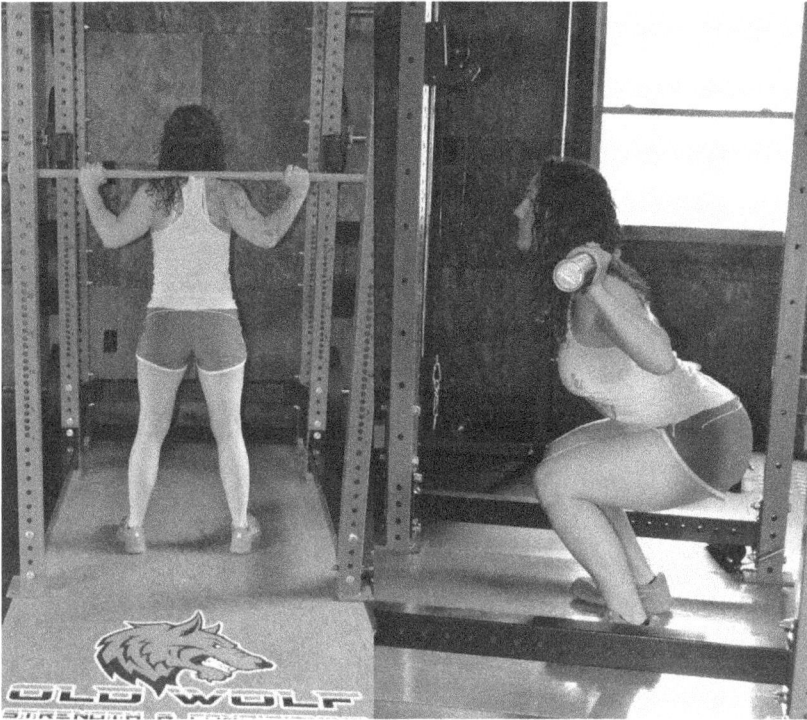

Figure 3.5. Squats. *Will and Renee Peveler.*

Leg Extensions

Leg extensions focus on the muscles of the quadriceps (rectus femoris, vastus intermedius, vastus lateralis, and vastus medialis). Before beginning leg extensions, ensure that the machine you are working on is set up specifically for you. Do not lock your knees out at the top of the knee extension.

Leg Curls

Leg curls are designed to strengthen the hamstrings (semitenndinosus, semi-membanosis, and biceps femoris). Because the gastrocnemius crosses the knee, it will be worked along with the hamstring muscles. Adjust the leg curl machine in accordance with the manufacturer's instructions. Leg curls (as well as leg extensions) are not typically recommended for sports performance because they are isolation exercises. However, muscular imbalances between quadriceps and hamstrings result in injury (primarily ACL injuries), so this exercise is important.

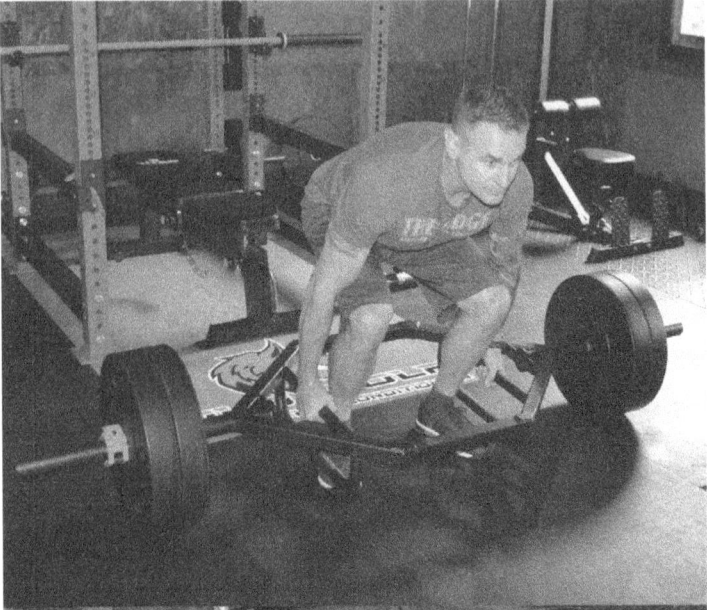

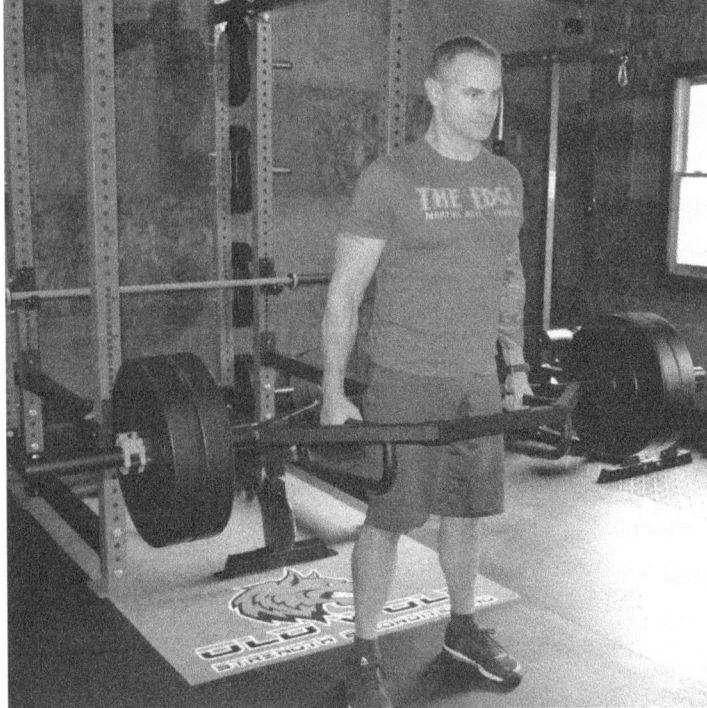

Figure 3.6.   Deadlift. *Will and Renee Peveler.*

Deadlift

The deadlift (see fig. 3.6) primarily focuses on the gluteus maximus, hamstring, quadriceps, erector spinae, rhomboid, and trapezius muscles. When conducting the deadlift, I recommend using a hex bar (trap bar) as opposed to a straight bar. When using a straight bar, you need to keep the bar as close to the shins as possible, which often leads to beat-up and gouged shins. The hex bar also puts your trunk in a more upright position and slightly reduces the risk of lower back injury. For those with lower back issues, most hex bars will have a higher handle that allows you to start from a higher position. Lastly, you are not competing in a power-lifting competition, and therefore a straight bar deadlift is not required. With the exception of slightly different knee angles and trunk angle, all other angles are the same and the work between a straight bar deadlift and a hex bar deadlift is the same (even though you can lift more with a hex bar). The center of gravity alters with a hex bar, and it allows for a more comfortable lift.

To conduct a hex bar deadlift, step into the hex bar with your feet about shoulder-width apart. Grab the bar and align it so that the center of the bar and center of the hands are at the midpoint of the ankle. When you grab the bar, do not bend at the waist and instead squat down. Drive the bar up from the feet and do not lift with the back. Thrust your hips forward as you come up (do not overexaggerate). During the eccentric phase (lowering back to the ground), make sure that the weights hit the floor evenly. If the weights touch the floor unevenly, you need to either slow down or drop weight in order to move smoothly through the motion so that both sides of the weight touch the floor at the same time.

Muscular Endurance Exercises

Pull-Ups

The pull-up (see fig. 3.7) is designed to improve the muscular endurance of the latissimus dorsi, teres major, and biceps brachii. The rhomboids are also worked when the shoulder blades are pulled together at the top of the pull-up. Grasp the pull-up bar a little wider than shoulder width with the hands facing away from you. In the start position, you will be hanging with your arms straight and no weight on the ground. Pull your body weight toward the bar until the chin clears the bar, and then return to the start position. Do not use a swinging motion during this movement. If you want to improve grip strength, you can do dial rod pull-ups or fingertip pull-ups.

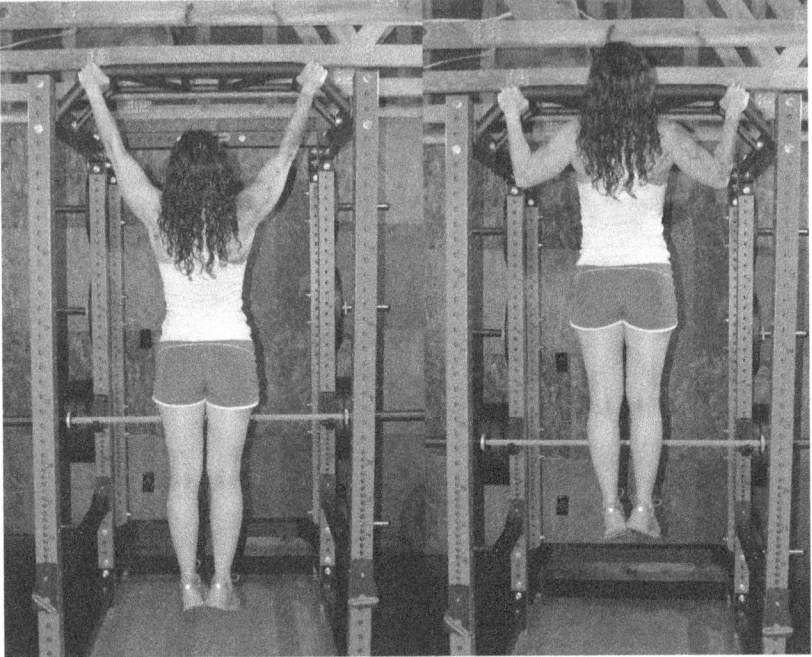

Figure 3.7. Pull-ups. *Will and Renee Peveler.*

Pull-ups are not easy, and it is quite common that beginners are unable to complete a pull-up. If you cannot complete a pull-up, there are methods to help you progress to that stage. One of those methods is the use of a lat pull-down machine. The muscles involved are the same, so as you increase your strength on the lat pull-down machine, you will increase your ability to conduct a pull-up. Another method is the assisted pull-up. In this process you will have some form of assistance to help during the pull-ups. Common forms of assistance are exercise bands, partner-assisted, and machine-assisted pull-ups. To use an exercise band, simply wrap the band around the pull-up bar and place a foot in the band. The elasticity of the band will assist as you pull up. With partner-assisted pull-ups, your partner will push your body weight up as you pull. Machine-assisted pull-ups require a specialized machine that uses weighted plates to help lift you as you conduct pull-ups. As you improve, you will reduce the amount of weight used to push you up during the pull-up.

Push-Ups

Push-ups are designed to increase the muscular endurance of the pectoralis major, anterior deltoid, and triceps brachii (see fig. 3.8). Lie facedown on the floor, placing your hands just wider than the shoulders. From this position, push up until the arms are straight. This is the start position. From the start position, lower your body until the elbows are approximately at a 90-degree angle, and then return to the start position. The weight should be borne by your hands and toes throughout the movement, and the body should stay straight. If you are just beginning, you can conduct a modified push by changing the contact point from your toes to your knees.

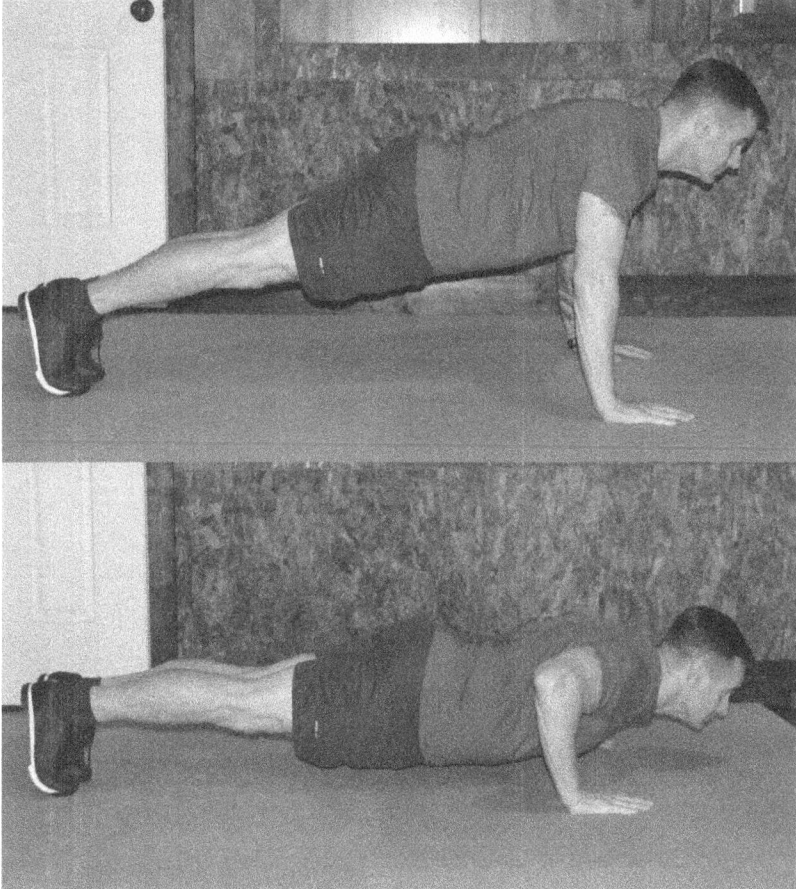

Figure 3.8. Push-ups. *Will and Renee Peveler.*

Dips

Dips are designed to primarily work the pectoralis major, triceps, and anterior deltoid. This movement is typically conducted on dip bars. Start with your arms at your side and extended at the elbow. Lower your body until your chest is even with the dip bars, and then push back up. You can alter the percentage of activation of the pectoralis and triceps by leaning your body. The more vertical you are, the more the triceps will be activated, and the more you lean forward, the more the pectoralis major will be activated (see fig. 3.9).

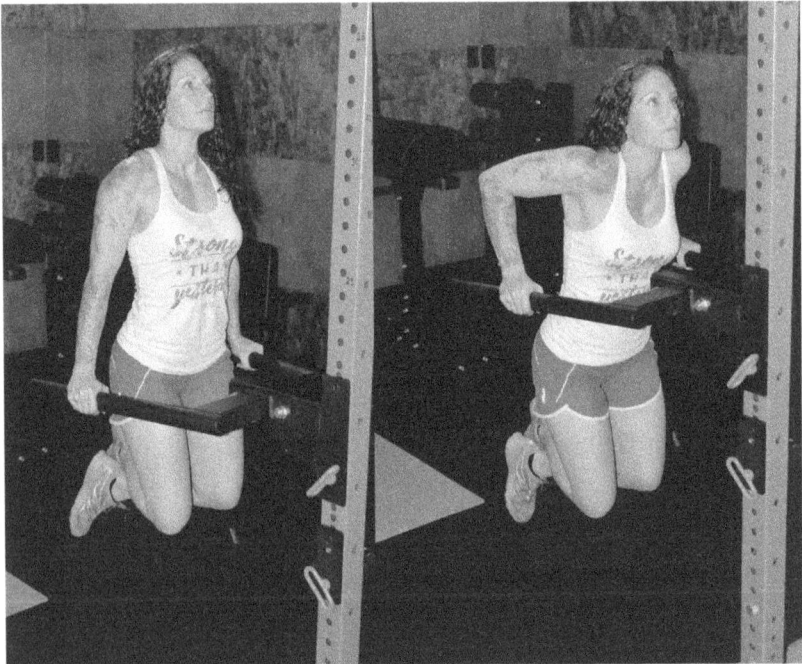

Figure 3.9. Dips. *Will and Renee Peveler.*

Horizontal Row

The horizontal row primarily focuses on the latissimus dorsi, rhomboids, trapezius, posterior deltoid, and biceps brachii. To conduct this exercise, you will need a horizontal bar (power rack and barbell will work) and a bench. From underneath, grab the bar with your hands a little wider than shoulder-width

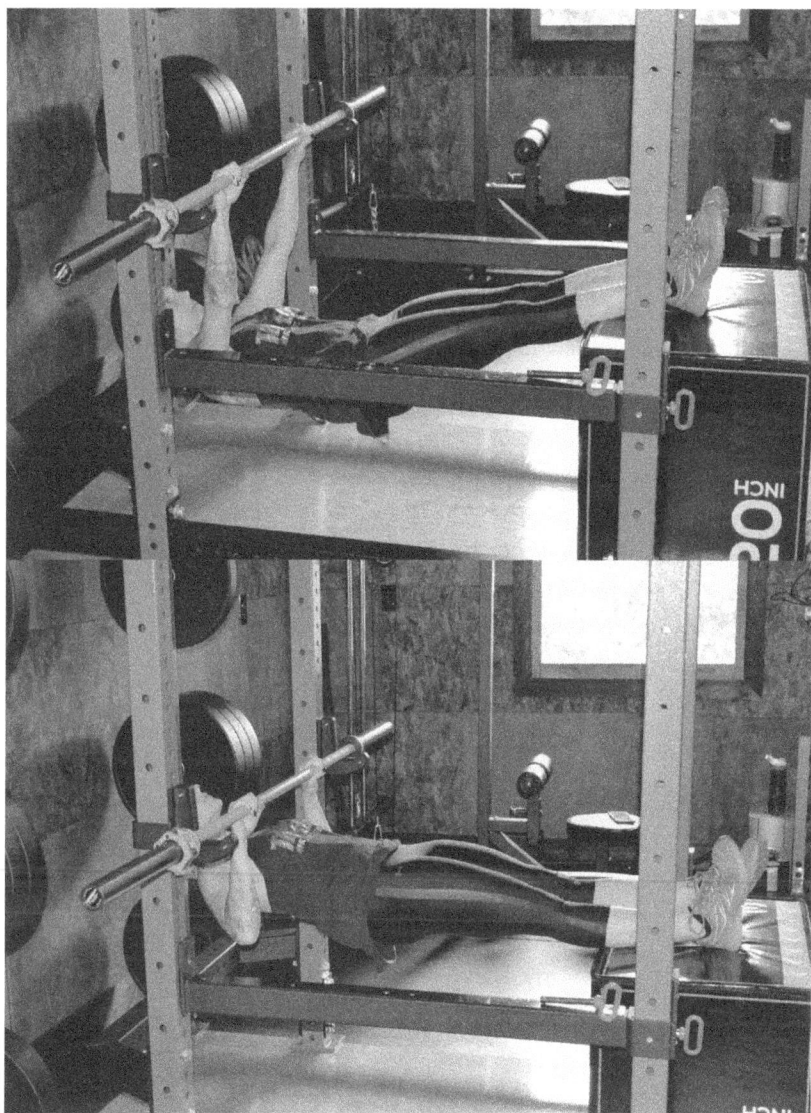

Figure 3.10. Horizontal row. *Will and Renee Peveler.*

apart and place your feet on the bench. Keeping your body in a straight line, pull up on the bar until your chest touches and then lower back down until your arms are straight (see fig. 3.10).

Lunges

The primary muscles involved in the lunge are the quadriceps, hamstrings, and gluteus maximus. Lunges can be conducted weighted or unweighted. Beginners should start by conducting lunges with no weights and progress to weighted lunges only when ready.

Start by placing your feet about shoulder-width apart. Step forward with your right leg and lower your body until the thigh of the right leg is parallel to the floor and the knee of the left leg is almost touching the floor. Return to the standing position and repeat this process by stepping forward with the left leg. Lunges can also be conducted in a walking manner by leaving the lead foot planted and bringing the rear leg forward into a lunge.

Army Crawl

When conducting the army low crawl (see fig. 3.11), lie prone with your weight on your forearms and lower body, and with your left knee bent and toward your left elbow. Move your right arm forward, and then push off with your left leg and bring your right leg up and your left arm up as your body moves forward. Repeat this process on the opposite side.

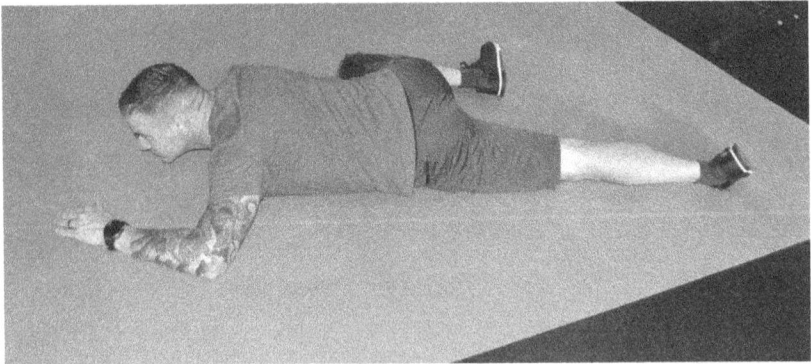

Figure 3.11.   Army crawl. *Will and Renee Peveler.*

Alligator Crawl

To conduct the alligator crawl (see fig. 3.12), begin in a push-up position. Bring your left leg toward and past your left elbow (on the outside of the arm) as you reach forward with your right arm while lowering your body almost to the floor.

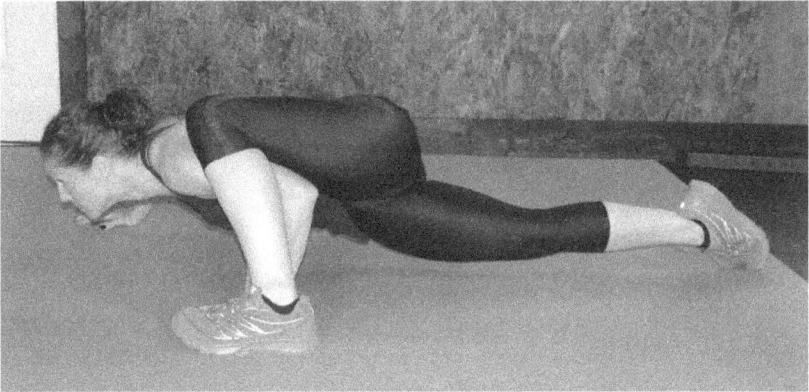

Figure 3.12. Alligator crawl. *Will and Renee Peveler.*

From this position you will push up as you lift your left hand and right foot. Move your left hand forward and your right knee toward and past your right elbow and lower to the ground as your left hand and right foot make contact. Repeat this process for the other side.

Bear Crawl

To conduct the bear crawl, position yourself with your hands, knees, and feet on the ground and your back straight and flat. To begin, lift your knees off the

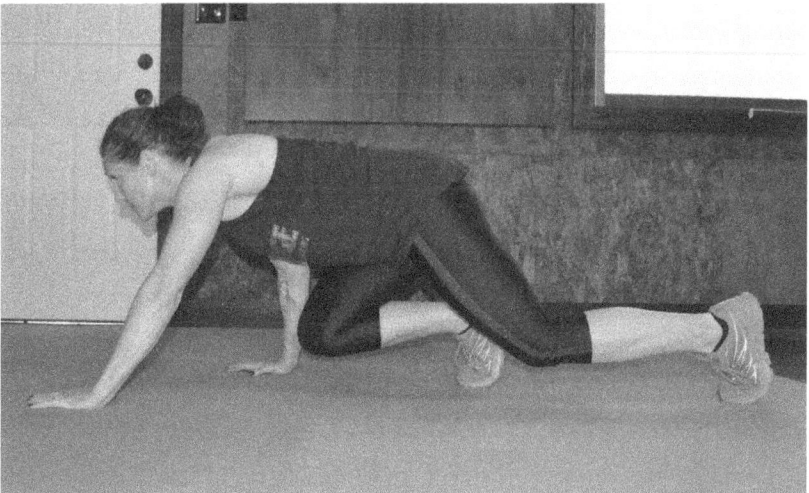

Figure 3.13. Bear crawl. *Will and Renee Peveler.*

ground to the point where your shins are about parallel to the floor and your back remains straight. Maintain a straight back and do not put your bottom high in the air. Walk by moving your left hand and right foot forward at the same time. You do not want to take large steps forward like you do with the alligator crawl. Instead, keep your legs basically in line with the arms. Repeat this process with the opposite leg and arm (see fig. 3.13),

Burpees

Burpees are not only a good exercise, but they are required in some obstacle course races. While I am listing burpees as a muscular endurance exercise, it can also be considered a plyometric exercise, due to the explosive nature. There are different variations to the burpee, but I am going to cover the basic exercise, shown in fig. 3.14. Begin with your legs slightly shoulder-width apart. Squat down, place your hands shoulder-width apart on the ground, and shoot your legs out to a push-up position. Next conduct a push-up, bring your legs back under you to the squat position, and jump high into the air. And then repeat.

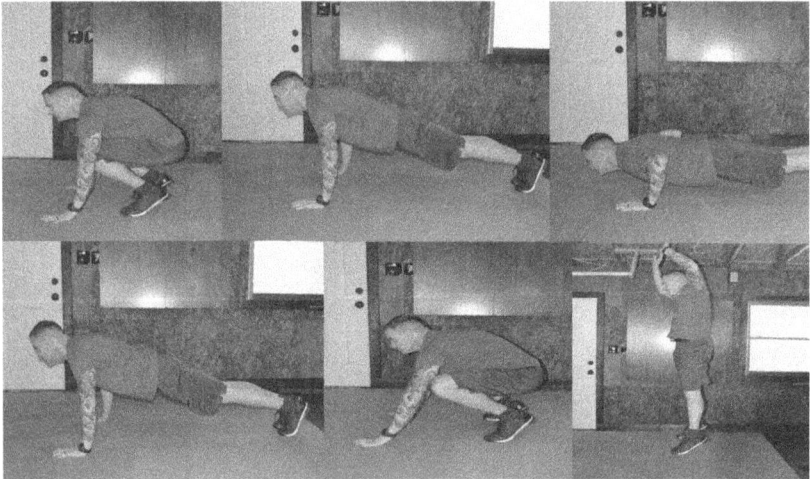

Figure 3.14.   Burpees. *Will and Renee Peveler.*

Core Exercises

There is a common misconception that the core muscles are primarily just the abdominal muscles and erector spinae muscles. However, the core is correctly defined as the multitude of muscles (approximately 29) that are designed to stabilize the pelvis and spine. The core muscles are worked during all the previously described lifting movements to stabilize the spine and pelvis throughout the lift. I am, however, going to describe common exercises that focus on the abdominals and the erector spinae. Those truly interested in developing a workout to develop core muscular endurance can expand this portion of their workout by adding more exercises.

Crunches

Crunches are designed to focus on the rectus abdominis and the oblique abdominals. Lie with your back on the floor and place your legs in the air, bending at the hips and knees. You can also conduct the crunch by placing your heels on a bench. Place your arms across your chest and curl your body off the floor until the upper back is clear of the floor. Repeat for as many reps as possible. After completing a set of normal crunches, you can add a set of twisting crunches. From the same start position, curl up, twisting your right shoulder to your left knee, and then return to the start position. On the next rep, curl up twisting the left shoulder to the right knee, and then return to the start position. Repeat this sequence until exhaustion.

Leg Raises

The leg raise is designed to work the abdominal and hip flexor muscles. Lie on your back with your head off the floor, arms at your side, and feet just off the floor. Lift your legs just past 90 degrees of hip flexion and then return to the start position. Keep your legs straight throughout this process.

Hanging Leg Raises

Hanging leg raises are designed to work the abdominal and the hip flexor muscles (see fig. 3.15). Hang from a bar or rings with your arms straight, and then curl up with your abdominal muscles as you bring your knees to your chest. You can twist to your left and right as you come up to focus more on the obliques.

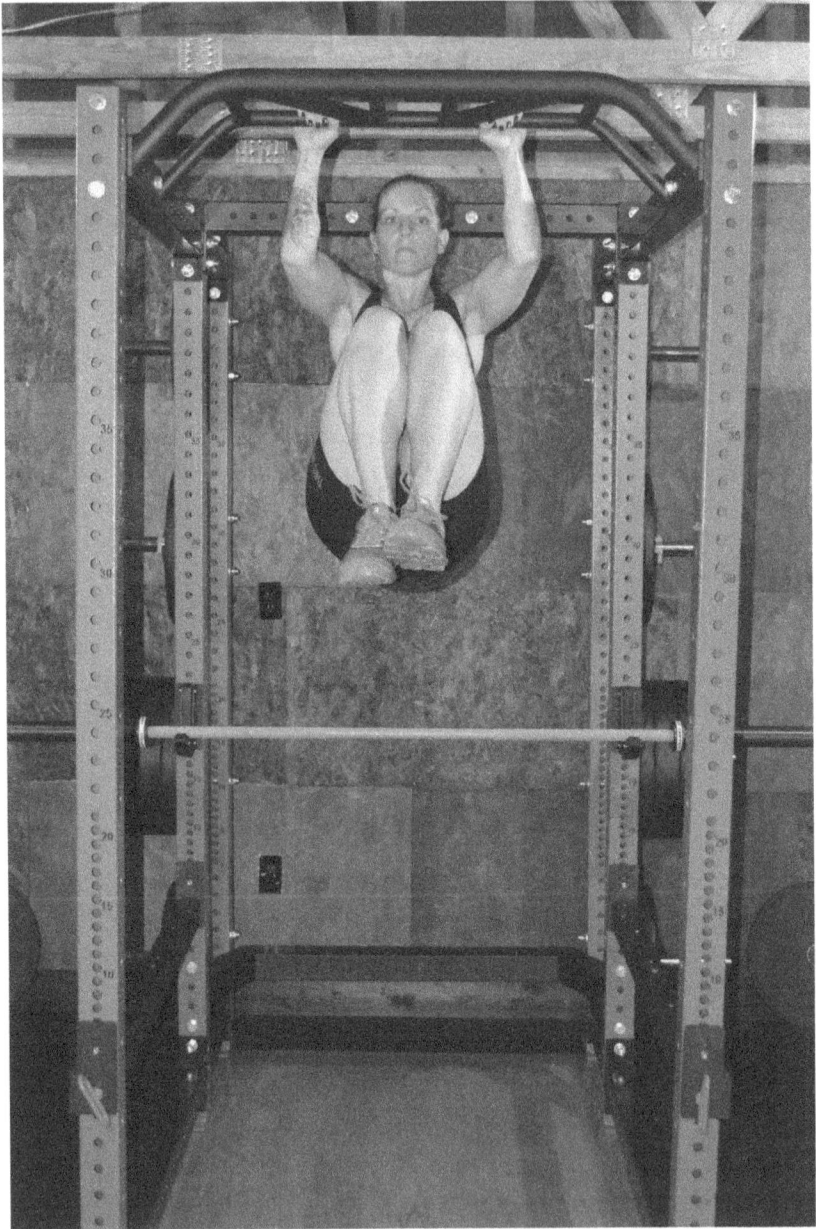

Figure 3.15.   Hanging leg raises. *Will and Renee Peveler.*

Roman Chair Back Extensions

The roman chair back extension works the erector spinae, glute, and hamstring muscles. Adjust the roman chair so that the ankles are under the pad and the thighs are on the support pads. Place your hands on or by your ears and bend forward at the waist and then extend your back upward (see fig. 3.16).

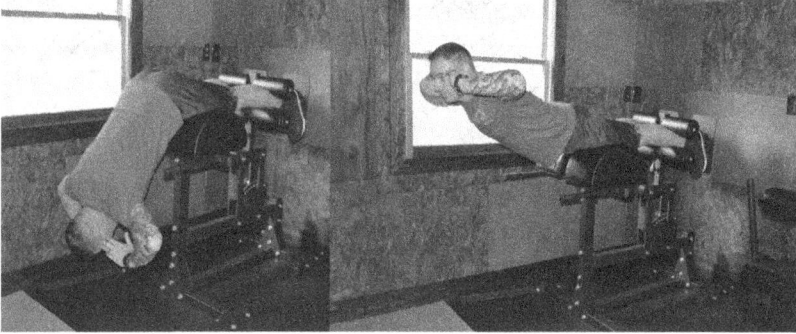

Figure 3.16.   Roman chair back extensions. *Will and Renee Peveler.*

Plyometrics

Plyometrics are a very important tool that will allow you to increase power upon completion of your strength-training phase. A plyometric exercise uses the stretch-shortening cycle to produce a more powerful movement. The stretch-shortening cycle involves an eccentric load that is stretched and then followed up by a powerful concentric contraction. An example of a plyometric movement is when you squat prior to a jump. When you squat down, you are stretching the eccentrically loaded muscles, and the concentric contraction occurs when you jump up from the squat. Adding in plyometrics will allow you to better utilize the stretch-shortening cycle to strike and move with greater power.

When adding in plyometrics, it is important to start slowly due to the heavy eccentric loads. As in all other workouts, make sure that you are using the correct techniques. Below I will discuss a few of the basic lower and upper body techniques that you can use in your training. There are many more valid plyometric exercises that can be used as well.

Box Jumps

When conducting box jumps (see fig. 3.17), choose a height that you can easily accomplish. While increasing height is how you will increase intensity, make sure that you can complete the desired number of repetitions prior to increasing height. Before beginning box jumps, I recommend conducting plyometric jumps from a flat surface. This will allow you to become accustomed to plyometrics before adding in the height of the box. Any jumps that you can do on the box, you can also do without a box. If you choose to purchase a plyometric jump box, I suggest buying a foam box as they are more forgiving on your shins than metal or wood boxes.

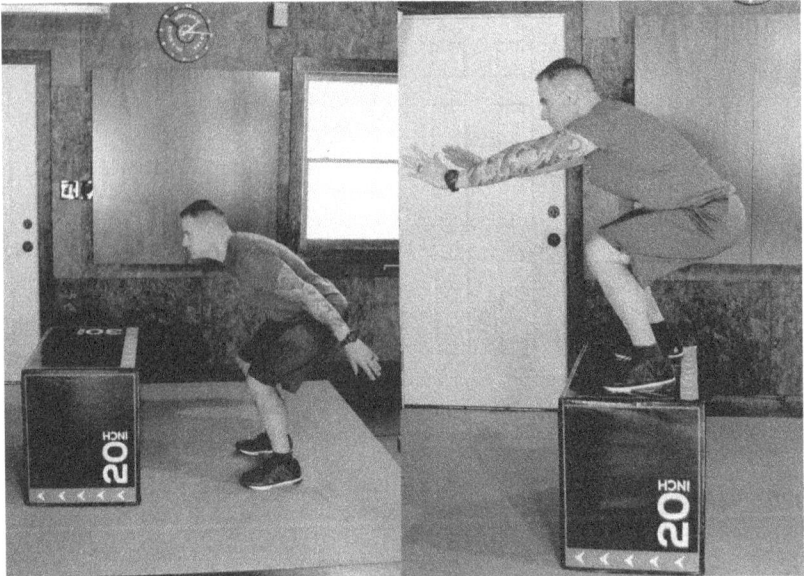

Figure 3.17.   Box jumps. *Will and Renee Peveler.*

Begin by standing close enough to the box that you can easily make the jump, and place your feet about shoulder-width apart. Make sure that you have enough space so that you do not hit the box on the way up. Squat down, moving your arms behind you (countermovement), and then jump up, landing with both feet in the center of the box. Next, jump down and then repeat. If you want to increase the workout, you can add a depth jump when you step off the box. To add the depth jump, step off the box, land on both feet, squat down, and jump again. Each of these movements should be completed in a controlled and fluid motion.

Lateral Box Jumps

Begin by standing next to the box so that your left side is facing the box. Make sure that you are close enough to the box to easily make the jump, but far enough away so that you do not hit the box on the way up. Squat down moving your arms behind you (countermovement), then jump laterally landing on the box. Step down on the opposite side, and then repeat the process going the other way (see fig. 3.18).

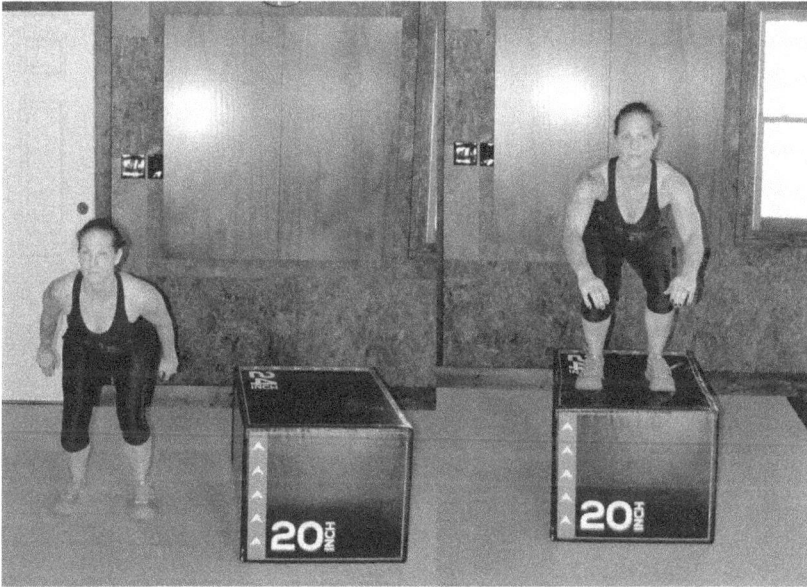

Figure 3.18.   Lateral box jumps. *Will and Renee Peveler.*

Chest Pass

When conducting upper body plyometrics, the use of a plyometric ball provides an optimal workout. Plyometric balls, also referred to as slam balls, wall balls, and medicine balls, come in different weights and different styles. Some balls are made to bounce, while others are made to minimize bounce. All types work, and you will need to find which you prefer. Plyometric balls come in different

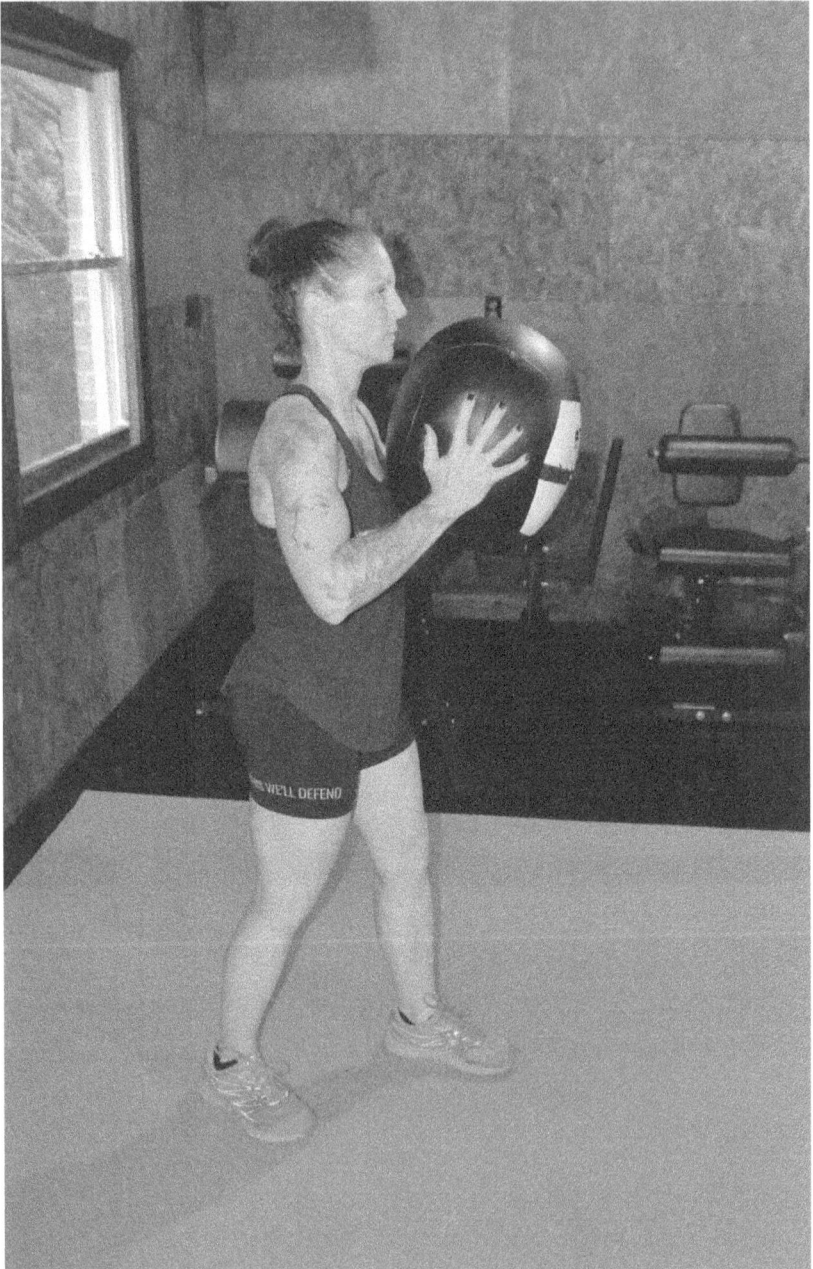

Figure 3.19. Chest pass. *Will and Renee Peveler*.

weights, so choose a weight that allows you to complete the desired repetitions, while maintaining correct technique.

The chest pass (see fig. 3.19) can be conducted individually or with a partner. If you are conducting the chest pass individually, find a wall that will not be damaged when the ball makes contact. If working with a partner, your partner will catch the ball and then chest-pass it back to you. If the weight of the ball makes it difficult for your partner to safely catch, then take turns on a wall.

Begin by placing your feet about shoulder-width apart. Bring the ball to your chest, creating the eccentric load, and then push the ball away in a quick concentric contraction. If you are working with a partner, you will use the eccentric load from the catch in order to immediately pass the ball back to your partner.

Side Throw

Begin by standing in an athletic stance with your left foot forward and facing the wall. Hold the plyometric ball in both hands and twist to the right, creating the eccentric load. Follow up with a strong concentric contraction, and release the ball as you twist to the left. Repeat this process for the opposite side of the body (see fig. 3.20).

Overhead Slam

Begin by placing your feet about shoulder-width apart. Bring the ball above your head, creating the eccentric load. Next, contract concentrically to slam the ball into the floor. You may want to choose a non-bouncing plyometric ball for this exercise. A plyometric ball that bounces can easily bounce up and hit you in the face. On the other hand, if you are careful, you can use a bouncing plyometric ball and catch it on the way back up as opposed to picking up a non-bouncing ball off the floor for every repetition (see fig. 3.21).

Squat Throw

Begin by placing your feet a little wider than shoulder-width apart. Squat down with a plyometric ball in both hands and between your legs, creating the eccentric load. Drive through your heels and upward with your legs as you bring the ball up with your arms until your arms are above your head. Release the ball so that it is over your head and flying behind you after release (see fig. 3.22).

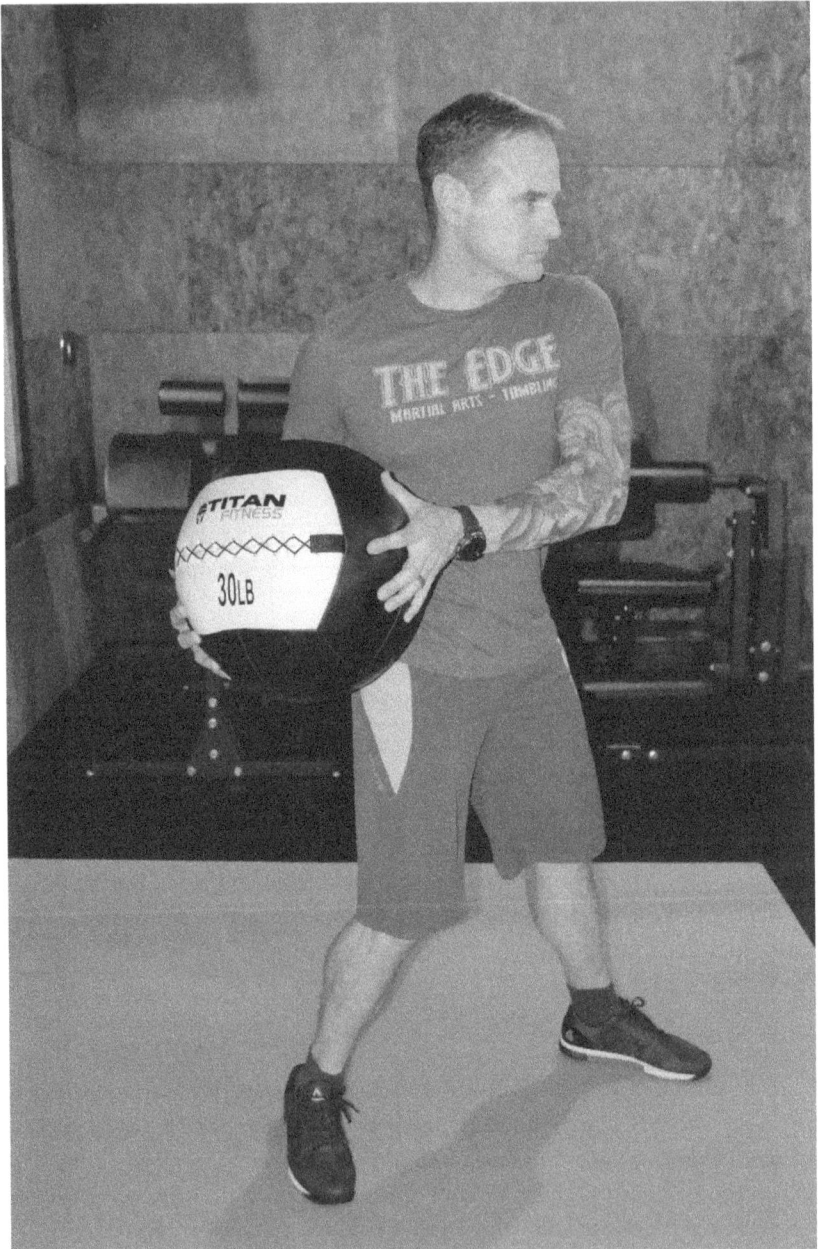

Figure 3.20.   Side throw. *Will and Renee Peveler.*

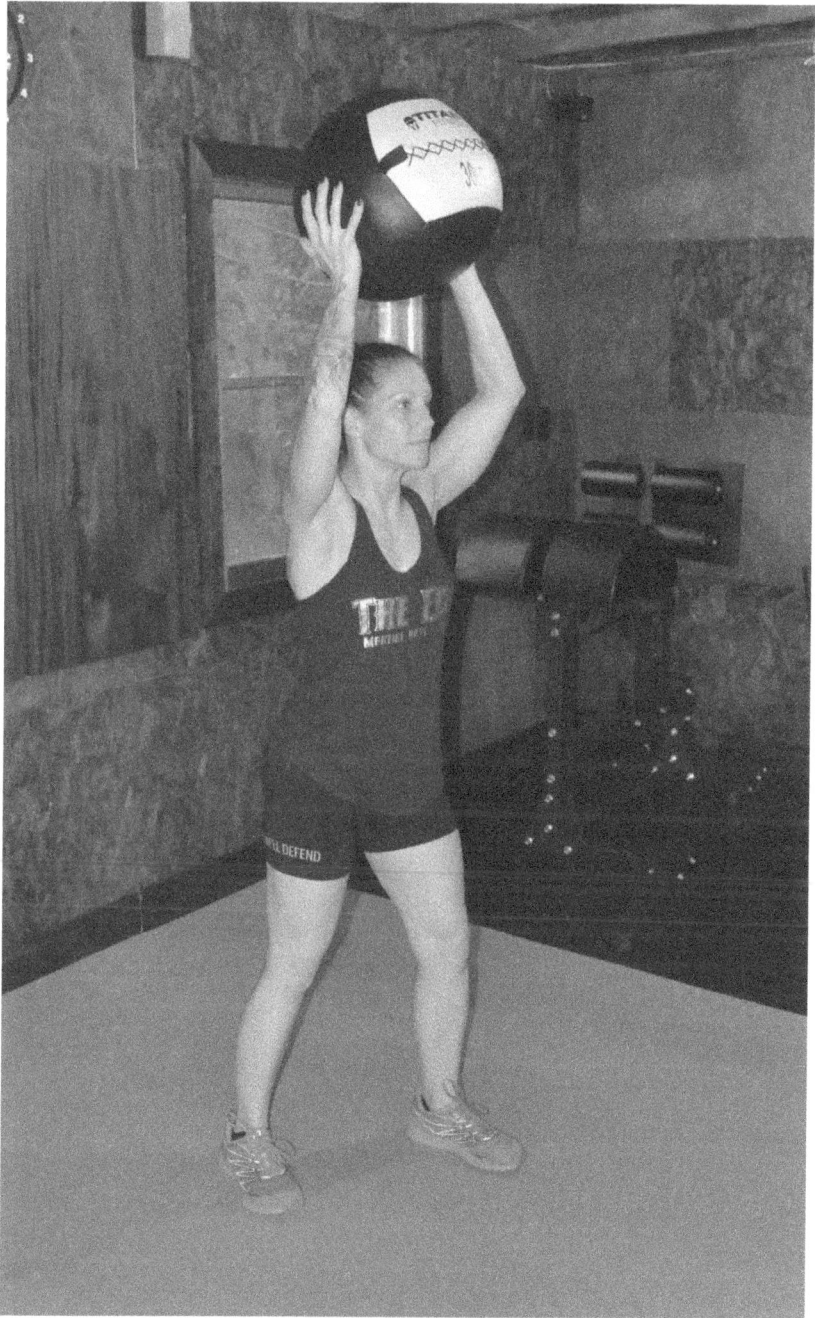

Figure 3.21. Overhead slam. *Will and Renee Peveler.*

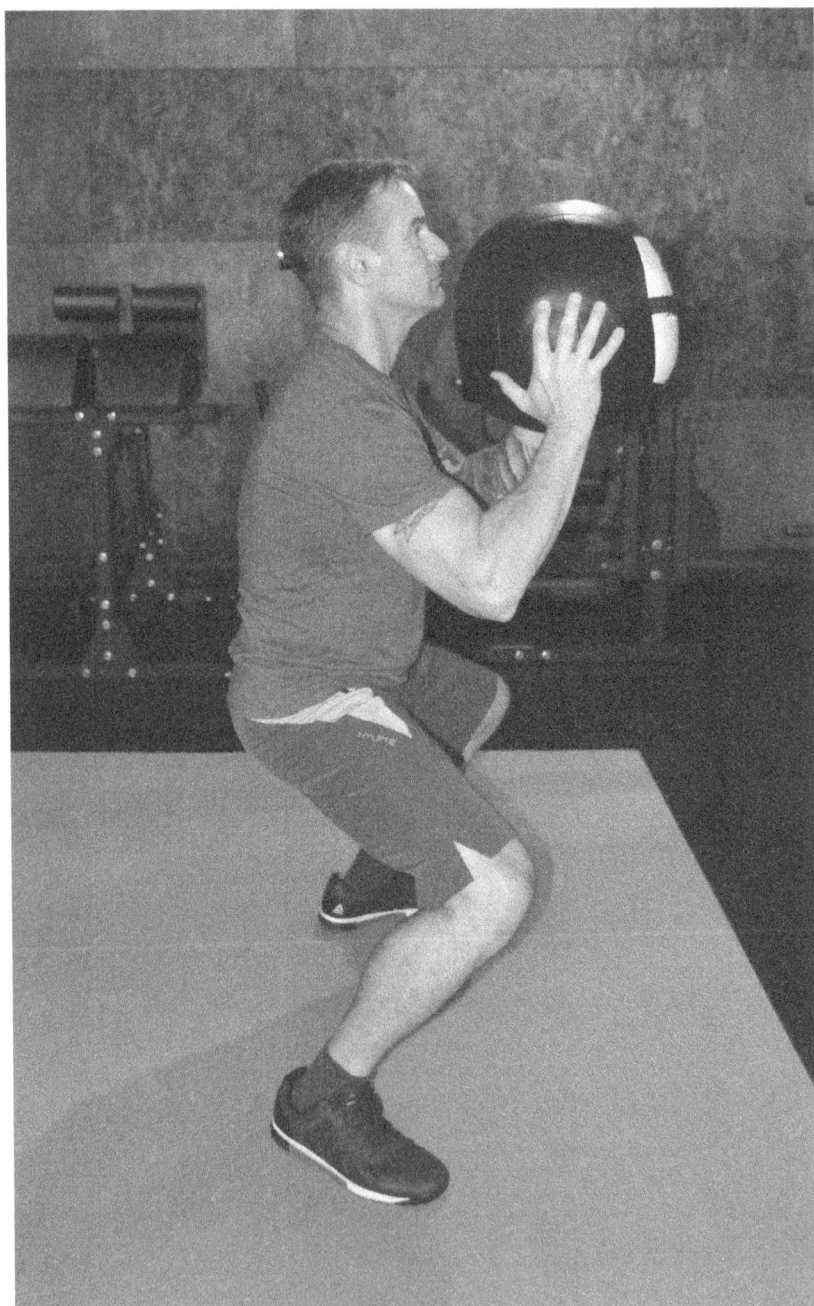

Figure 3.22.   Squat throw. *Will and Renee Peveler.*

Stair Workouts

Stair workouts can be done to increase power, aerobic capacity, anaerobic capacity, or a combination of the three. As obstacle course races are never flat, these workouts can provide significant improvements in performance. If you choose to add a stair workout to your program, keep these factors in mind. When stairs are run at a slow pace that you can handle, it will be more of an aerobic workout. However, for most individuals, if you are running stairs, it will be at a higher intensity and therefore it will be an anaerobic workout. Keep in mind that plyometrics are still involved, but not optimized during the anaerobic workout. In order to make it a plyometric workout, decrease your speed and focus on the plyometric aspects; for example, instead of running, you could double leg hop, single leg hop, etc., at a slow pace.

When conducting stair workouts there are a few things to keep in mind. The first is that stairs are constructed of hard material and are very unforgiving on the body. Always proceed carefully. Make sure that your shoes are tied securely prior to beginning your session, and check periodically throughout. Keep your focus on your technique throughout the exercise, and if you become too fatigued to maintain proper technique, then quit for the day. Most accidents occur because the athlete becomes too fatigued to conduct the movement, a foot catches, and they fall.

FLEXIBILITY

Flexibility is your ability to move each joint through the complete range of motion for that particular joint. Maintaining a dynamic range of motion and proper flexibility is very important for obstacle course racing. However, flexibility is often overlooked by many athletes, resulting in decreased performance and overuse injuries.

There are different methods used to increase flexibility. However, this book will only focus on the two primary methods and when to use them. The first method used to increase flexibility is called static stretching. When conducting a static stretch, slowly move into the proper position for that specific stretch and hold it for 30 seconds. When you move into the stretch, only go to the point of slight discomfort. Never go until you feel pain as it is counterproductive, causing the muscle to tighten during the stretch.

The second method of stretching I recommend is dynamic stretching. This method will require that you move through the full range of motion for a particular joint in a dynamic manner without holding a stretch. Dynamic stretching is used during warm-ups for competition in order to increase range of motion and optimize performance.

Both static and dynamic stretching have a place in your training and competition. There is currently debate on whether static stretching is harmful prior to competition. Some research states that power and speed are reduced when static stretching is used, as opposed to dynamic stretching. However, the current pool of research is not conclusive. I would recommend dynamic stretching going into your competition and training, and static for after. Static stretching is key when it comes to increasing range of motion and should remain an integral part of your training program.

Flexibility Exercises

Neck Stretches

When stretching the muscles of your neck it is important to include rotation, flexion, extension, and lateral flexion.

- Begin by rotating your head to the left as far as it will turn and hold, then repeat this process to the right.
- Take your neck into flexion by trying to touch your chin to your chest and hold the stretch. Next move your head into extension by rotating your chin toward the ceiling and hold.
- Take your head into lateral flexion to the right by taking your right ear toward your shoulder. Hold that position, and then repeat this process to the left.

When stretching the neck, it is very important to not apply a large force or to conduct these movements in a fast or bouncing manner.

Anterior Shoulder Stretch

This stretch is designed to stretch the anterior deltoid and pectoralis major. Raise your arm until it is parallel to the floor and place your hand on any object that will not move (such as a wall, door frame, etc.). Next rotate your upper body away from the arm that is being held in place, stretching the anterior muscles of the shoulder.

Posterior Shoulder Stretch

The posterior shoulder stretch focuses on the posterior deltoid and muscles of the back. Horizontally draw your right arm across the chest, then place your left hand on the elbow and apply pressure to stretch.

Behind the Head Stretch

This stretch focuses on the triceps and latisimus dorsi. Raise your right arm above your head, and then flex at the elbow until your hand is behind your head. Reach up with your left hand to grab your elbow and apply pressure to the left. Repeat this process with the left arm.

Abdominal Stretch

As the name indicates, this stretch will focus on the abdominal muscles. Lie prone and place your hands palm down on the floor. Push upward with your arms, leaving your lower body flat on the floor.

Lower Body Exercises

Calf Stretch

The calf muscle (triceps surae) is made up of the gastrocnemius and soleus muscles. To stretch the calf muscle, stand on a raised surface with the fore part of your foot on the surface and the heel hanging off the surface. Allow your heel to go down by placing the foot in dorsiflexion. To concentrate on the gastrocnemius, keep the leg straight during this process. To focus more on the soleus, slightly flex at the knee and repeat the process. Placing the knee into flexion places slack on the gastrocnemius and allows a greater focus on the soleus. This is important because even at the bottom of your pedal stroke your knee is flexed.

Hamstring Stretch

The basic hamstring stretch does much more than just stretch the hamstrings. This stretch is also great for the muscles of the lower back. If you can reach your toes and pull the foot into dorsiflexion, it will also stretch the calf. While this stretch can be conducted standing, I advise conducting the stretch seated. Sit with your legs together and straight out in front of you. Bend forward at the waist, going as far forward and down as possible. Grab your toes and pull the foot into dorsiflexion. If you cannot reach your toes, grab as far down the leg as you can. During this process, keep your legs straight and do not allow a lot of bend at the knee.

Modified Hurdle Stretch

The modified hurdle stretch (see fig. 3.23) primarily concentrates on the hamstrings and muscles of the lower back. Sit on your bottom with your left leg straight out in front of you and your right leg flexed at the knee with the bottom of your foot in contact with your left leg. Bend forward and attempt to place both hands on your left foot. Repeat this stretch with the right side.

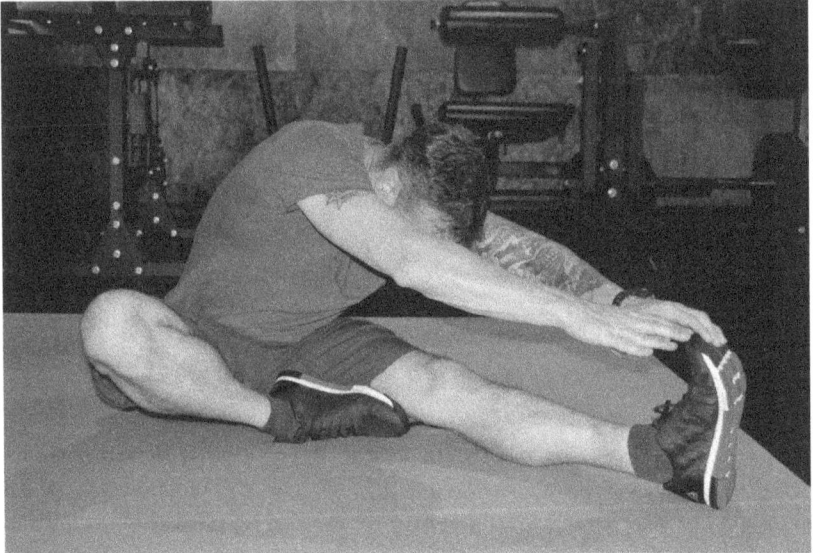

Figure 3.23. Modified hurdle stretch. *Will and Renee Peveler.*

Straddle Stretch

This stretch primarily focuses on the hamstrings, adductor muscles, and muscles of the lower back. Sit on your bottom with your legs spread wide (horizontal split). Lean your body over your left leg, attempting to touch your foot with your right hand, and then repeat the movement on your right leg. Once you have completed those movements, bend toward the floor in the middle.

Quadriceps Stretch

The quadriceps stretch is typically conducted incorrectly by trying to push the heel into the gluteus maximus while in flexion. Instead, reach behind your body and grab your right leg with your left hand, then place the knee into flexion and pull rearward. Repeat this process with the other leg. If you have trouble balancing on one leg during this process, move to a wall and place your free hand on the wall for balance.

Adductor Stretch

The adductor stretch (butterfly stretch) focuses on the adductor muscles. Sit on the floor and place your knees into flexion with the soles of your feet touching. Grab your feet and place your elbows on your legs. Push down on your legs with your elbows and bend forward at the waist.

Hip Stretch

This stretch concentrates on the gluteus maximus and hamstrings. Lie supine with both legs straight out. Bring your right leg up by flexing at the hip. As you bring the leg up, allow the knee to go into flexion. Place your hands behind the knee and pull. Repeat this process with the left leg.

Supine Twist

This stretch focuses on muscles around the spine, the external oblique and gluteus muscles. Lay on your left side, keeping your left leg straight and bending your right knee. Your left arm should be perpendicular to your body and laying on the ground with your right arm on top of the left. Keeping your right leg in place, rotate your upper body toward the right, placing your shoulders flat on the ground; your right arm should now be on the ground and perpendicular to your body. Repeat this process on your right side.

Dynamic Stretches

Wrist Rotations

Wrist rotations are conducted by rotating both wrists clockwise for about 15 seconds and then reverse to counterclockwise for another 15 seconds.

Cross-Body Arm Swings

To conduct the cross-body arm swings, horizontally abduct your arms and then adduct them across your chest with one arm slightly above the other as they cross. Alternate which arm is above and below with each swing.

Elbow Circles

With arms slightly raised from your sides, make circles from the elbow. You will not actually have rotation at the elbow, it will be more like circumduction with slight shoulder movement. Start by going counterclockwise for 15 seconds and then clockwise for another 15 seconds.

Arm Circles

Rotate your arms from the shoulders in a 360-degree circle (circumduction). Conduct arm rotations to the front for 15 seconds, and then rotate them to the back for 15 seconds.

Trunk Rotation

Place your feet a little wider than shoulder-width apart and abduct your arms until they are approximately parallel to the floor, then rotate as far as you can go to the left and then back as far as you can go to the right.

Butt Kicks

Butt kicks can be conducted in place, or while walking or jogging. As your foot comes off the ground, drive the heel to your butt with each step. Alternate legs as you perform the dynamic stretch. When you first start this movement, your heel may not reach your butt. This is okay, just get your heel as high as you can.

High Knees

High knees can be done in place, or while walking or jogging. When the foot leaves the ground, bring your knee as high as possible toward your chest. Alternate legs as you do this dynamic stretch.

High-Knee Hip Circles

Conduct this movement in place. Bring your knee up high toward your chest and then rotate the leg away from your body and then back to the ground landing in your starting position. Alternate legs as you conduct this movement. After 15 seconds reverse this movement (rotate from the outside in).

Leg Swings

You can conduct leg swings with or without support. If you need support for balance, place your hand on a wall or non-moveable object. Without bending your knee, kick your leg forward as high as possible and then allow it to swing down and behind you as far as possible. After 15 seconds switch to the other leg and conduct leg swings for another 15 seconds.

Lateral Leg Swings

Lateral leg swings are similar to leg swings, but instead of front to back you will swing your leg from side to side (abduct and adduct). Kick your leg to the side, and then allow it to come down and cross in front of your stationary leg. After 15 seconds switch to the other leg and conduct leg swings for another 15 seconds.

Supine Leg Circles

To conduct supine leg circles, lay on your back and bend at the hips until your thighs are perpendicular to the floor and then move your feet in circles. Move your left foot clockwise and your right foot counterclockwise. After 15 seconds reverse each foot for another 15 seconds.

4

DEVELOPING A
TRAINING PLAN

The previous chapters of this book discussed basic training principles, basic physiology, basic psychology, and areas of training for obstacle course racing. These chapters are important because they provide important foundational information that will help you to build a solid training program. Before you can build an optimal program, however, you must have a strong foundation of knowledge. In this chapter, I am going to discuss how to develop a strong training program built around the demands of your everyday life.

When developing your program, there are a few key points to remember. The first is that more than one road exists, and there are many different paths to your destination. Do not get too caught up on designing the perfect program in your first attempt. Design a sound program and make changes as you go based on marked improvements in performance and monitoring adaptation. Keep in mind that as long as you are not overtraining, you are fine. Do not be afraid of making a mistake when developing your program, because you will. Just learn from those mistakes and improve. Understand that your strength-and-conditioning program is an evolving and learning process.

Another key point is to stick with your program. While you do want the program to evolve with your progression, you do not want to move away from the key training principles, which are the foundation of program development. The key training principles will always remain true. One of the biggest mistakes beginners make is that they quit a program before the training has an opportunity to elicit a positive change, and then just jump from program to program with no real gains. Develop a sound program and stick with it. You will need to make alterations to volume and intensity based on how your body responds to the stimulus, but the program itself does not change.

Start small and work your way up to the appropriate volume. Trying to do too much too soon will lead to overuse injuries and maladaptation. Slowly add to your volume, and only add intensity when you have developed a sound endurance base. The two most common mistakes beginners make here are to train at maximal intensity every time they train and to train too often, not allowing time for recovery. It is important to develop a training program that integrates the hard and easy principle discussed in chapter 2, and to stay within the assigned intensity parameters for that particular training session. It is also vital that you incorporate dedicated recovery days into your training program.

The last key point is to write everything down as it avoids random disorganized training. This is especially true when trying to work a training program into your everyday life. If you do not schedule and make your training a priority, then things will get in the way and you will keep putting your training off and then have no time to complete it. Take the time and effort to write out your program as it provides a clear map toward your desired goals. When you write your training program down, you are more likely to follow the plan. It is also a good idea to record your progression as well, as this allows you to track your short-term goals.

There are three common approaches to developing a training program. The first involves hiring a coach to help you develop and implement a training program. The second is to use a boxed training plan from an online website or a book. The last approach involves creating your own training program, which is what this book is designed to help you do. I will, however, also speak on the first two approaches.

COACHING

In Person

If you are serious about obstacle course racing, I recommend that you hire a qualified coach to help you achieve your goals. Look for a coach with documented coaching experience and a background in exercise science. You want a coach who can develop a sound program and understand the physiological mechanisms behind training and training adaptations. You should also consider the coach's experience as a racer. Coaches with race experience will have a better understanding of what it is like to compete in obstacle course racing and therefore can provide meaningful feedback. However, it is important to note that how fast a coach is when he races has no bearing on his ability to coach. I have known many elite athletes who could not put together a sound training program.

If you are going to hire a coach, it is vital that you find a qualified coach. To better assess a coach's abilities, interview the athletes that he is currently coaching as well as athletes he has coached in the past. Check for any coaching certifications or formal education.

Often coaches will have certifications in strength and conditioning as well. The most widely respected strength-and-conditioning certification is the National Strength and Conditioning Association Certified Strength and Conditioning Specialists (CSCS). This certification requires the coach to possess a four-year degree, pass a rigorous certification exam, and supply continuing education credits after obtaining the certification.

While hiring a coach is ideal, it will require an ongoing budget to pay coaching fees. Not only do you need to research the coaches' credentials, but it's also important to compare fees among different coaches to determine your cost-to-benefit ratio. Keep in mind that like most things in life, you get what you pay for. If you choose to hire a coach, it is one of those areas that you may not want to skimp on.

Online

Online coaching is another option and has become very popular in recent history. With current technology, a coach can work with you online and never even meet with you face-to-face. Many modern watches contain a GPS and heart rate monitoring, which allow coaches to evaluate performance, mark adaptations, and prescribe training based on those adaptations. Modern technology makes online coaching a viable option. Prior to committing to an online program, examine all coaching level options, pricing, and reviews.

Online boxed training plans are another option. These training plans provide a day-to-day generic training plan without the interaction of a coach. Boxed plans use a "one size fits all" approach to training. There are no variations to these programs as everyone receives the same package. You will receive weekly training plans to use to improve your performance, but you will receive no coaching or advice on how to alter the program to elicit optimal adaptations.

These rigid programs are designed to provide lower volumes and intensities so that the average person can increase performance while ensuring overtraining does not occur. A boxed training program can be useful for beginners as it provides a safe, structured place to begin training. However, if you want to excel at obstacle course racing, you will need to make adaptations to the training plan based on your progression and how your body is adapting to the training volume and intensity.

DEVELOPING A TRAINING PROGRAM

The previous chapters of this book provide you with the foundations needed to develop a strong program. This chapter provides the necessary steps. When developing your own program, you must take into account your current fitness level, obstacle course racing experience, work schedule, and family schedule. Developing a program for the first time can seem overwhelming, and it can easily become frustrating. Just like anything else in life, it is important to start the journey by mapping it out and then taking your first step. The information below will give you a generic outline to use and adjust to your specific needs. As you become more advanced, you can alter the program to keep up with your advancements.

Determine Goals

The first step in this process is to determine your goals. It is important to set challenging but realistic goals based on your current fitness level, prioritization of obstacle course racing, and available time to train. If you have never raced before, ensure that you give yourself plenty of time to train prior to your first race. On a piece of paper, write out the following questions and answer them:

- What is my overall goal for obstacle course racing? (List all goals.)
- What is my current fitness level?
- What is my current skill level for each obstacle?
- How much time can I devote to training?
- What are my logistical challenges?
- What is my racing and training budget?

After answering the questions, set both short- and long-term goals. Your original list of goals will most likely all be long-term goals. Examples of long-term goals may be to participate in a race, lose weight, or become healthier and more active. For each of those long-term goals, set short-term goals. Look at it like a ladder. If you only had the bottom and top rungs of the ladder, you would be unable to climb to the top (your long-term goal). You need to add rungs to the ladder (short-term goals) in order to reach the top. Short-term goals give you easily reachable goals to strive for. If you have a long-term goal of racing a 13-mile obstacle course race but have never raced before, then you should set short-term goals to help you reach that long-term racing goal. Your first short-term goal may be to train for and compete in a 3- to 4-mile obstacle course race and build from there. You would then develop a program that slowly increases distance and intensity over time until you are able to reach your long-term goal of a 13-mile obstacle course race.

Write down both your long- and short-term goals in your training log so that you have them for future reference. It is important to record your goals as writing them down makes it more likely that you will actively pursue them. Making a short list of goals and posting it somewhere you will see them on a regular basis will help to keep you motivated.

Baseline Measures

At the start of your program you should be recording baseline measures, which will allow you to mark the start of your journey and then to measure improvements in performance. It also gives you an unbiased look at your current fitness and skill levels.

Baseline measures can be either conducted in a laboratory setting or in a field setting. Lab-based measures are conducted in an environmentally controlled setting using precise measurement techniques and laboratory equipment. Some of the common lab-based tests are: $VO_{2\,max}$ testing, threshold testing, and body composition. While lab-based tests are excellent for providing baseline measures and for marking progression, they may not be readily available in your area and may not be cost-effective.

Often field-based methods are used in place of lab-based methods due to the ease of conducting the tests. Field-based tests do not require special training or expensive equipment and are extremely easy to conduct and analyze. They can often be conducted at no charge as well.

Time trials are the most commonly used field-based tests used to conduct baseline measures for aerobic and anaerobic performance. A time trial requires that you run as fast as you can over a fixed distance. Treat the time trial as though it were a race. Make sure that you are well rested and well hydrated prior to conducting a time trial session. Also make sure that the weather is not too hot, too cold, or too windy when conducting your time trial.

To conduct an aerobic time trial, pick your desired distance and running course. Choose a distance that is representative of the distance you plan to race, such as 5 km for a short obstacle course race. To measure anaerobic performance, choose a 400-meter track as it will provide a flat and reliable course. While you can opt for shorter or longer distances (no longer than 800 m), 400 meters is a solid measure of your anaerobic performance.

You can repeat the time trial session periodically throughout your training season in order to determine whether your program is working. Conduct the time trial on the same course and under the same conditions. You cannot compare times from one running course to another as every course is different. If your times continue to improve throughout the season, then you know that your program is working well. If there is no perceivable change or if times get worse, you should examine your training program.

You should also set baseline measures for your muscular endurance for the various obstacles that you may encounter. As there are a lot of overhead obstacles, pull-ups are a great way to monitor your muscular endurance. Keep in mind that most people cannot perform a large number of pull-ups, if any, when they begin. Do not get discouraged, and continue to work toward your goal. Or if you have access to overhead obstacles, see how many times you can go back and forth without falling. Monkey bars at your local park will work for this test. You can also conduct bucket carry, rope climbing, and many other obstacles as a baseline measure for obstacle course racing. Once you establish your baseline measures, you can periodically retest to determine if your program is producing the results you are striving toward.

Determine Volume

Your training volume will be determined by the frequency and duration of your training sessions. Training volume can be calculated by a single session, as a weekly schedule, or as a multiweek time period. Your actual training volume will be determined by the desired training goal of the training phase you are currently in. When training for obstacle course racing, your overall volume will include both your cardiovascular training and your resistance.

When determining your training volume, there are two primary factors to consider, the first of which involves how much time you can dedicate to your training. Determine how many days a week you can train, how many training sessions per day, and how much time per session you can dedicate. Due to your individual responsibilities, you may be limited on the number of days a week you can dedicate to training. The second concern deals with the prescribed training volume for that particular training phase, which will fluctuate throughout your training season and will be determined by the specific goal of that training phase.

In order to determine which days during the week you have available for training and the time slots available on those days, write out your weekly schedule. Include your work hours as well as any other recurring commitments. This process will give you a realistic idea of how much time you can devote to training. The allotted time slot should be large enough to not only accommodate actual training time but also logistics such as travel time, prep time, and cleanup.

You should train a minimum of three days per week. However, if you want to excel at obstacle course racing, then you should train at least five days per week. Advanced racers can train six to seven days per week if they correctly implement recovery training within the training schedule. You may need to conduct two different training sessions within one day (two-a-day): endurance training in one session and resistance training in a second session. Be cautious when implementing two-a-day training sessions as they will result in overtraining if not correctly applied.

You must also determine the duration of each training session. The duration will be highly dependent on the goal of that day's training session and your current fitness level. For example, if your scheduled run is a long, slow distance session, then the duration could be 13 miles if you are an advanced racer or 3 miles if you are just starting out. If you are running trails, you may want to consider using time as opposed to distance in order to determine duration as the terrain varies from trail to trail. You would be able to complete a 5-mile flat course much faster than you could a 5-mile course with large elevation changes. Whereas, if you are scheduled to run 45 minutes, then you can run 45 minutes on a flat trail or a hilly course and it is 45 minutes either way.

The volume for your resistance training sessions will be determined by the sets and repetitions for each exercise. In previous chapters I discuss numerous exercises for resistance training. Do not attempt to insert all the exercises listed previously into your training program all at once as the volume will be too high. The exercises are listed and explained so that you may choose those you want to implement into your program. These exercises are designed to achieve specific goals, and you must make sure that the exercises you choose are designed to align with your training goals for that particular phase.

Training sessions do not have to be long in order to be effective. Many resistance training sessions will be under an hour. Combined training sessions (endurance and resistance training) will typically be around one to two hours, depending on the focus of each session. While you want to include travel time, changing time, social time, etc., into your daily time schedule, do not include those factors when evaluating training volume. Just include the time frame from the start to the finish of your training session.

Determine Intensity

Once you have determined your overall training volume, you will need to determine intensity. When determining the training intensity for endurance training, keep in mind the hard–easy principle, and make sure that you are not training too hard too often. Choose your training zone based on the training goal for that day (recovery, aerobic, threshold, or interval). Unless your periodization block requires high intensity for that time period, do not conduct more than two high-intensity sessions per week. You can do more if you are in a specific periodization program that permits a higher level of volume and intensity followed by recovery. Low-intensity days (recovery, aerobic) should be monitored and controlled using a heart rate monitor and defined training zones.

Intensity for your resistance training will be determined by the resistance chosen for each exercise. If you are using weights, then the intensity will increase as you increase the weight used. For muscular endurance, you typically work on just increasing volume (number of repetitions), but you can increase intensity by adding weight to your body when conducting muscular endurance exercises. Beginners can begin at lower intensities by decreasing their body weight during muscular endurance exercises. For example, if you cannot conduct pull-ups, then attach a resistance band to the pull-up bar and place one foot in the band in order to reduce the effect of your body weight and make the pull-ups easier to accomplish. Another example of lowering intensity for muscular endurance is to perform push-ups on your knees instead of your feet in order to reduce the effect of your body weight.

Periodization

Periodization breaks up the training cycle into specific training periods, allowing the athlete to optimize performance. The human body is not designed to continually adapt to high-intensity levels and volumes without recovery. In other words, you cannot train at full speed year-round without allowing for recovery. By breaking your training into specific cycles, you optimize both stimulus and recovery periods. The idea of periodization is to develop a training plan that allows the athlete to alter training intensity and volume in order to peak during the season with mini peaks throughout the season in order to optimize performance at key competitions. When looking at periodization, there are three primary levels: macrocycle, mesocycle, and microcycle. I will first discuss each level of periodization, and then I will provide example training plans.

Macrocycle

The largest of these cycles is called the macrocycle, and for most traditional sports it covers a year of training (preseason, in-season, and off-season). For OCR, the macrocycle will be divided into 3 distinct phases: preparation (often called preseason), in-season, and off-season. To develop your macrocycle, determine the dates of your first and last planned races for the upcoming year. While obstacle course races occur throughout the year, the primary race season runs from March to October. After determining the length of your season, you will then divide the season into your 3 phases. It is okay to race year-round as long as you do not try to peak for the off-season races. As an aside: You can race year-round and divide your year into macrocycles where you peak for specific races throughout the year as long as you work recovery phases into the macrocycle. This method takes more detailed planning than what I cover in this book, however.

Preparation. The first of the three phases is the preparation phase, which is commonly known as the preseason. The preparation phase will typically last 9 to 12 weeks but can be longer or shorter depending on how important your first races are. During the preparation phase you will focus on increasing volume and intensity, building up to the in-season phase. During this phase you will work on increasing your volume first in order to provide a strong base. Once volume has sufficiently increased, you will begin increasing intensity. The beginning, middle, and end of the preparation phase is a good time to conduct physiological testing (time trials, $VO_{2\,max}$, etc.) in order to ensure optimal training and adaptations. Your preseason numbers should be lower than both your previous race season numbers and your upcoming season numbers. So, do not be stressed if your runs are a little slower. An exception to this rule is if you were working to improve a specific aspect over the off-season, for example, if you were weak during the overhead obstacles and wanted to focus on increasing your upper body muscular endurance in the off-season. In this case, if your off-season workout program was successful, then you should have higher numbers for your upper body muscular endurance tests.

In-Season. The in-season phase is commonly referred to as the race season. You will need to establish all the races in which you would like to compete in order to develop your mesocycle (explained below) so that you peak optimally for your key races.

Off-Season. The off-season phase serves two main purposes. First, it allows for a decrease in volume and intensity, which helps you to recover both physically and mentally from the race season. Racing places a heavy toll on your physical and mental capacities, and it is easy to become burned out if you do not plan a recovery period. Second, it allows you to not only decrease volume and intensity but also to alter training in order to perform better the following season. Implementing an off-season resistance program, while maintaining an aerobic base, is key to performance improvements the following season. Seasons can be won or lost depending on your off-season training program. The length of the off-season can vary between 6 and 10 weeks based on the length of the race season in your area and your desired length of the following preparation phase.

A typical macrocycle for OCR would be in-season from April to October, off-season from November to January, and preparation from February to March. The yearly macrocycle could shift depending upon how you set up your race season. Once you determine your in-season, you can adjust the off-season and preparation phases.

Mesocycle

The mesocycle is a sub-cycle of the macrocycle and typically covers approximately a four-week period of training, but can range anywhere from one to eight weeks. There are multiple phases that can be used within a mesocycle, which can alter depending on the specific goals of that cycle. You will design your mesocycle so that the training program will alternate volume and intensity by increasing the stimulus to the point at which you will peak so that your performance peaks at the appropriate time. After the peak you will have a brief recovery period followed by increased stimulus toward another peak.

Common phases in a mesocycle are the preparation phase, build phase, peak/competition (taper occurs in this phase), recovery, and transition. You will need to develop mesocycles for your competition, off-season, and preparation macrocycle phases. During the preparation phase, more focus is placed on increasing volume as opposed to increasing intensity. The build phase is designed to increase intensity, which will in turn increase anaerobic threshold and improve race performance.

Tapering occurs after the build phase, allowing the body to recover from the previous stages in order to optimally perform for the upcoming race. Depending on the event, tapering can last one to two weeks. A one-week taper is sufficient for most events. Tapering for a race is often misunderstood and therefore conducted incorrectly. Often athletes will cut their volume and intensity too much or for too long a period of time, resulting in suboptimal performance come race day. When tapering, slightly decrease overall volume seven days prior to the event as well as reduce training intensity and the number of high-intensity days. The two days before the race should be very easy days, nothing hard or long.

Your training will peak at the competition phase. You can schedule your mesocycle to peak for one race or for multiple races. If you plan to peak for multiple races, do not attempt to hold that peak for more than two to three weeks before moving to a recovery phase.

A one- to two-week recovery phase will follow the competition phase. The recovery phase is vital as it permits your body to fully recover for competition and to move into the next preparation phase leading up to your next race. This phase will have a slightly lower volume and intensity. If it is the last competition phase of the race season, then you will transition into the off-season.

In order to set up your mesocycles effectively, first determine your race schedule for the upcoming season. Choose your races, and prioritize them as A (top priority), B (medium priority), or C (low priority). You should schedule your mesocycles so that you peak for all A races. Peaking for a B race is nice but not a priority, and C races are typically considered training races. It is common for many obstacle course racers to compete in running races between scheduled obstacle course events. This is a good practice but must be put into perspective when planning your schedule. These races should be used as training races as opposed to A-level races if your primary goal for the season is obstacle course racing. Now that you have your races scheduled and prioritized, develop your mesocycles to peak at the appropriate times.

If you can travel easily or if you have a number of races to choose from within your local area, you can actually do the reverse of this process. Set up your mesocycles evenly spaced and then pick races that occur when you naturally peak in your designed mesocycle.

Table 4.1 shows an example of a mesocycle where the first priority race occurs eight weeks into the race season. In this example, there is one C-level race prior to the first A race. You will treat the C race as a training race. You can conduct a mini taper if you'd like or just incorporate the race into your training schedule as a hard day. Your training program for week 9 will depend on your race schedule. If you don't have another A race within the next three weeks, schedule a recovery week and go right back into another preparatory phase. If you have another A race within the next three weeks, then schedule a couple

Table 4.1. In-Season Mesocycle Example with a C-Level Race Prior to an A-Level Race

April				May			
In-Season							
Week 1	Week 2	Week 3 C Race	Week 4	Week 5	Week 6	Week 7	Week 8 A Race
Preparation Phase			Build Phase				Taper and Race

days of recovery time and then maintain the peak until after the next A race. Then roll into another mesocycle.

The mesocycle for your preparation phase (preseason) will be slightly different than that of your in-season as you will most likely have no preseason races, and if you do, those races should be considered more for fun and training as opposed to placement. If it is an important race, then adjust the dates of your off-season and preseason in your macrocycle so the race is within the season and you peak for that race. During the preseason, you will spend the first part of the season in the preparation mesocycle to focus on increasing your training volume. Remember that your training volume decreases significantly in the off-season. The second mesocycle in the preseason is the build phase where you will focus on increasing intensity while maintaining your volume built during the preparation phase (see table 4.2).

During the off-season you will decrease your overall volume and intensity. Keep in mind that the off-season is not sitting on the couch, watching TV, and counting down to your preseason. While your overall volume and intensity will drop, there will be areas that you will focus on improving during this time. In those areas you will have a preparation and a build phase. Implementing an off-season resistance focus is recommended as it will also improve your endurance performance in the upcoming season. As a point of interest, off-season

Table 4.2. Off-Season Mesocycle Training for Increasing Intensity

February				March			
Preparation Phase (Preseason)							
Week 1	Week 2	Week 3	Week 4	Week 5	Week 6	Week 7	Week 8
Preparation Phase				Build Phase			

resistance training does improve endurance performance, but does not improve aerobic capacity. Instead, improvements will come from neuromuscular adaptations. Off-season training can also focus on areas of weakness (muscular strength, muscular endurance, muscular power, etc.).

The following tables provide off-season mesocycles. While not shown, you would have a one- to two-week transition period in October. Use that transition period to recover physically and mentally from your race season. Keep in mind that the preparation phase will typically include increases in volume and the build phase will focus on increases in intensity. You will peak at the end of each phase in the off-season, but it will not be a performance peak. Instead, it will be a peak in volume or intensity for that portion of training. The breakdown of endurance versus resistance training will not be evident until you plan the microcycle. The off-season with four mesocycles is shown in table 4.3, and the off-season with six mesocycles is shown in table 4.4.

You can also have a phase that will focus on a specific area of training. For example, you can focus a six-week preparation and six-week build phase on

Table 4.3. Off-Season Training with Four Mesocycles

November				December				January			
Off-Season											
Week 1	Week 2	Week 3	Week 4	Week 5	Week 6	Week 7	Week 8	Week 9	Week 10	Week 11	Week 12
Preparation Phase		Build Phase				Preparation Phase				Build Phase	

Table 4.4. Off-Season Training with Six Mesocycles

November				December				January			
Off-Season											
Week 1	Week 2	Week 3	Week 4	Week 5	Week 6	Week 7	Week 8	Week 9	Week 10	Week 11	Week 12
Preparation Phase		Build Phase		Preparation Phase		Build Phase		Preparation Phase		Build Phase	

Table 4.5. Off-Season Training with Focus on a Specific Area of Training

November					December				January		
Off-Season											
Week 1	Week 2	Week 3	Week 4	Week 5	Week 6	Week 7	Week 8	Week 9	Week 10	Week 11	Week 12
Preparation Phase						Build Phase					

resistance training while maintaining your endurance volume and intensity at a normal off-season level (table 4.5).

Microcycle

Now that you know the overall training goals (macrocycle) and have divided those goals into purposeful training periods (mesocycle), the next step is to determine your weekly training schedule. The microcycle is the weekly training program where you schedule the day-to-day training. While a microcycle typically covers the full week, you can break it down into smaller microcycles within a week time period when needed.

When developing a microcycle for obstacle course racing, you must often schedule multiple types of training. At times you will schedule endurance training and resistance training on the same day. The ideal way to accomplish this would be to conduct both within the same time block instead of splitting the training into two separate sessions. This allows for better recovery for your next training day. However, you may not have a two-hour block to train during the day and may need to divide your training into two training sessions (two-a-days). When conducting all your training within one block of time, decide which is the more important focus of the day, endurance or resistance. Whichever activity you do first will negatively impact the second. If you are conducting two-a-days, the effect on the second training session will be less than if they were conducted within the same block, and the second training session of the day will give you less time to recover before the following day. And finally, if possible, attempt to train at approximately the same time every day to allow close to 24 hours of recovery between bouts.

Below are three examples of weekly training plans for a microcycle for the in-season for beginners. The first two examples (tables 4.6 and 4.7) are

Table 4.6. In-Season Weekly Microcycle Training Plan 1 for Beginners with Resistance and Endurance on the Same Day

Day	Monday	Tuesday	Wednesday	Thursday	Friday	Saturday	Sunday
Training	Recovery	Recovery	Resistance Mid-Distance Run, Zone 3	Recovery	Recovery	Resistance Long-Distance Run, Zone 2	Resistance Long-Distance Run, Zone 2

Table 4.7. In-Season Weekly Microcycle Training Plan 2 for Beginners with Resistance and Endurance on the Same Day

Day	Monday	Tuesday	Wednesday	Thursday	Friday	Saturday	Sunday
Training	Resistance Long-Distance Run, Zone 2	Recovery	Resistance Mid-Distance Run, Zone 3	Recovery	Resistance Long-Distance Run, Zone 2	Recovery	Recovery

Table 4.8. In-Season Weekly Microcycle Training Plan for Beginners with Resistance and Endurance on Different Days

Day	Monday	Tuesday	Wednesday	Thursday	Friday	Saturday	Sunday
Training	Resistance	Long-Distance Run, Zone 2	Recovery	Resistance	Mid-Distance Run, Zone 3	Long-Distance Run, Zone 2	Recovery

Table 4.9. Off-Season Weekly Microcycle Training Plan for Advanced Cyclists

Day	Monday	Tuesday	Wednesday	Thursday	Friday	Saturday	Sunday
Training	Resistance	Medium-Distance Run, Zone 2	Resistance Intervals	Recovery Run, Zone 1	Resistance Run, Zone 3	Long, Slow Distance Run, Zone 2	Recovery Run, Zone 1 or Day Off

Table 4.10. Off-Season Weekly Microcycle Plan for Resistance Training

Day	Monday	Tuesday	Wednesday	Thursday	Friday	Saturday	Sunday
Training	Resistance Training	Medium-Distance Run, Zone 2	Resistance Training	Recovery Run, Zone 1	Resistance Training	Long-Distance Run, Zone 2	Recovery

designed with both resistance and endurance training completed on the same day, which can be as a single session or as individual two-a-day sessions. The third example program (table 4.8) shows resistance and endurance training on separate days. The first weekly training plan has you training three days a week with four recovery days during the week. This allows you to get in the minimum training to complete a race while not interfering too much with the workweek. The second beginner program has the same volume but leaves your weekends free. Keep in mind that this is a beginner program designed to get you started.

Table 4.9 is an example of a more advanced weekly training plan. This plan has you working six to seven days during the week, depending on whether or not you take Sunday off. Recovery runs need to be low mileage and easy within zone one. If you go too hard or too long, it is no longer a recovery day and will negatively impact your training and gains. If possible, conduct the Wednesday and Friday workouts as one session. On Wednesday, conduct the intervals after the resistance training. Friday can be conducted as either resistance first or run first.

For off-season training, the microcycle will be highly dependent upon what you are focusing on improving. The resistance training in a microcycle schedule for the off-season (see table 4.10) can focus on muscular endurance, muscular strength, muscular power, or a combination of any of those. This will also change depending on your goal. Your off-season can flow from a strength focus to a muscular endurance focus to a power focus as you are coming into the preseason. Or you could just focus on one or two of those areas in the off-season.

The following tables show examples of daily routines for off-season resistance training. Table 4.11 provides a minimal resistance plan focused on muscular strength; table 4.12 is an example of an in-depth resistance training program focused on muscular strength; table 4.13 is an in-depth resistance training program focused on muscular endurance; table 4.14 shows a resistance training program focused on muscular power; and table 4.15 provides a resistance training program focused on both muscular endurance and muscular strength.

Table 4.11. Daily Routine for Off-Season Resistance Training: Minimal Resistance Plan Focused on Muscular Strength

Exercise	Sets	Repetitions
Bench Press	3	6–8
Lat Pull-Down	3	6–8
Squats	3	6–8
Crunches	3	Assigned Number or Volitional Exhaustion
Back Extensions	3	Assigned Number or Volitional Exhaustion

Table 4.12. Daily Routine for Off-Season Resistance Training: In-Depth Resistance Training Program Focused on Muscular Strength

Exercise	Sets	Repetitions
Bench Press	3	6–8
Overhead Press	3	6–8
Lat Pull-Down	3	6–8
Squats	3	6–8
Deadlifts	3	6–8
Calf Raises	3	6–8
Crunches	3	Assigned Number or Volitional Exhaustion
Back Extensions	3	Assigned Number or Volitional Exhaustion

Table 4.13. Daily Routine for Off-Season Resistance Training: In-Depth Resistance Training Program Focused on Muscular Endurance

Exercise	Sets	Repetitions
Push-Ups	3	Assigned Number or Volitional Exhaustion
Dips	3	Assigned Number or Volitional Exhaustion
Pull-Ups	3	Assigned Number or Volitional Exhaustion
Horizontal Rows	3	Assigned Number or Volitional Exhaustion
Burpees	3	Assigned Number or Volitional Exhaustion
Alligator Crawls	3	Assigned Number or Volitional Exhaustion
Lunges	3	Assigned Number or Volitional Exhaustion
Crunches	3	Assigned Number or Volitional Exhaustion
Back Extensions	3	Assigned Number or Volitional Exhaustion

Table 4.14. Daily Routine for Off-Season Resistance Training: Resistance Training Program Focused on Muscular Power

Exercise	Sets	Repetitions
Box Jumps	3	Assigned Number or Volitional Exhaustion
Lateral Box Jumps	3	Assigned Number or Volitional Exhaustion
Chest Pass	3	Assigned Number or Volitional Exhaustion
Overhead Slam	3	Assigned Number or Volitional Exhaustion
Squat Throw	3	Assigned Number or Volitional Exhaustion
Crunches	3	Assigned Number or Volitional Exhaustion
Back Extensions	3	Assigned Number or Volitional Exhaustion

Table 4.15. Daily Routine for Off-Season Resistance Training: Resistance Training Program Focused on Both Muscular Endurance and Muscular Strength

Exercise	Sets	Repetitions
Push-Ups	3	Assigned Number or Volitional Exhaustion
Dumbbell Press	3	8–12
Pull-Ups	3	Assigned Number or Volitional Exhaustion
Seated Rows	3	8–12
Deadlifts	3	8–12
Lunges	3	Assigned Number or Volitional Exhaustion
Crunches	3	Assigned Number or Volitional Exhaustion
Back Extensions	3	Assigned Number or Volitional Exhaustion

You can also add rope workouts, stadium stair workouts, and obstacle-specific workouts to this list. For obstacle-specific workouts, add the rope climb, overhead obstacles, and bucket carry exercises. As most of your upper body obstacle work will require pulling, make sure that you have an adequate number of pushing workouts in your training plan as well.

Conduct muscular endurance sessions that will solely focus on obstacles you will commonly encounter when racing. This will be interchangeable with the "resistance" marked in the microcycle above. You could do two days with muscular endurance and one day with obstacle-based muscular endurance, two days of obstacle-based muscular endurance, or all days of obstacle-based muscular endurance. This ratio can change depending on where you are in your macrocycle and mesocycle. For an example plan for obstacle-specific training, see table 4.16.

Table 4.16. Example Plan for Obstacle-Specific Training

Exercise	Sets	Repetitions
Push-Ups	3	Assigned Number or Volitional Exhaustion
Rope Climbs	3	Assigned Number or Volitional Exhaustion
Bucket Carry	3	Assigned Number or Volitional Exhaustion
Tire Flip	3	Assigned Number or Volitional Exhaustion
Monkey Bars/Rings	3	Assigned Number or Volitional Exhaustion
Burpees	3	Assigned Number or Volitional Exhaustion
Alligator Crawls	3	Assigned Number or Volitional Exhaustion
Sled Pull	3	Assigned Number or Volitional Exhaustion
Crunches	3	Assigned Number or Volitional Exhaustion
Back Extensions	3	Assigned Number or Volitional Exhaustion

TRAINING LOG

Throughout the process of creating your training program, it is vital that you put your plan into writing by developing a training log. The training log has multiple purposes that will assist in your training and progression. The first purpose of a training log is to give you a detailed road map to follow. You will know exactly what the daily workout routine will be and will stay focused on your goal and not get sidetracked.

The second benefit is that it will keep you motivated. Research has shown that if you write out your plans in detail, you will be more likely to follow those plans. On days that you may not feel like working out, it will provide that little push to get you going. It helps with accountability.

The third major benefit is that recording your daily workouts allows you to monitor your progression. Improvements in performance occur slowly over time, and often we do not recognize these improvements. Looking back in your training log will help you to assess your progression in a quantitative and detailed manner.

Developing Your Training Log

As your training log will be specific to your individualized program, it would be difficult to find a preprinted training log that would specifically fit your needs. Luckily with today's technology, creating your own training log with all the specifics you need is very simple and affordable. I will provide key criteria to use when developing your training log. Do not put so much information in your log that it becomes overwhelming and useless. You will need the following information when developing your log:

Date and Time. Record the date and time of the workout for future reference to look for patterns in your training and progression.

Body Weight and Body Fat Percentage. Tracking body weight serves two main purposes: to monitor alterations to body weight over time and to track fluid loss when training in the heat in order to optimize rehydration. When possible, measure body weight before every training session, and after a training session as well when training in the heat. Body fat percentage allows you to examine fat and fat free mass over a period of time but does not need to be done every training session.

Morning Heart Rate. Check morning heart rate to determine readiness for training; an increased morning heart rate over consecutive days could indicate overtraining or dehydration. It also allows you to record adaptations to endurance training as morning heart rate will decrease over time with training.

Type of Training. State the type of training conducted: muscular endurance, muscular power, endurance training, etc.

Volume. For cardiorespiratory training, record the distance and time of the session. For resistance training, record the sets and reps for each exercise. And for anaerobic training, record the time, sets, and distances.

Intensity. Record all measures (HR, RPE, weight, etc.) used to determine intensity during the training session. Record time in and time out of the desired training zones when appropriate.

General Comments on the Training Session. General comments provide an opportunity to include other pertinent information (weather, fatigue, injury, sleep, stress levels, etc.).

5

NUTRITION

One of the most important components of an athlete's training program is nutrition. Too often athletes will spend a large amount of time developing and implementing a training program and yet completely ignore any form of nutritional planning. It is important to develop a nutritional plan that will optimize anabolic processes for recovery and provide adequate fuel for training and competing. The purpose of this chapter is to provide a basic introduction to nutrition in order to optimize OCR performance. The discussed guidelines are general in nature and designed for healthy individuals who do not have dietary restrictions. If you are regularly taking medication or have a known illness, check with your physician prior to altering your nutritional intake. If you have dietary restrictions, it is always a good idea to work with a registered dietitian who has a background in sports nutrition and can establish a detailed nutrition plan tailored to your specific needs and goals. Even if you have no dietary restrictions, working with a registered dietitian with a background in sports nutrition would be beneficial.

NUTRIENTS

There are six basic categories of nutrients that are important for athletic performance: carbohydrates, fats, proteins, vitamins, minerals, and water. These nutrients are responsible for everything from energy transfer to anabolic processes, and each plays a specific role in normal body function. Having a basic functional understanding of the specific nutrients, how they work, where they originate, and how they impact OCR performance will allow you to develop a rational and sustainable nutritional program.

Carbohydrates

Carbohydrates are one of the main fuel sources for the human body. Carbohydrates are ingested and then converted to glucose for transportation in the blood and glycogen for storage in the muscles and liver. Glycogen is not only important as fuel for athletic performance; it is also the only fuel source that the central nervous system and the brain can utilize. When glycogen stores become low during prolonged exercise, you become fatigued and confused. This is typically termed "bonking" and is often experienced during long endurance performances. The human body is limited to roughly 2,000–2,500 kCals of stored glycogen.

The daily recommended intake of carbohydrates will differ depending on volume of physical activity (athlete or nonathlete). For a nonathlete, roughly 50 percent of daily caloric intake should come from carbohydrates, as opposed to 60 to 70 percent of an endurance athlete's daily intake. To more precisely determine carbohydrate intake, the average individual should consume 5 to 6 grams of carbohydrates per kilogram of body mass per day, and endurance athletes should consume 7 to 10 grams per day. This range is highly dependent on the volume and intensity of training. As the training volume or intensity increases so too will the recommended intake.

For example, a 74.83-kg (165-lb) obstacle course racer would need to ingest between 523.81 and 748.30 grams of carbohydrates each day, depending on training volume and intensity. To give you an idea of what that looks like in food, a cup of plain oatmeal contains about 28 grams of carbohydrates, there are between 35 and 39 grams in a baked potato, and a small serving of pasta will contain about 40 to 50 grams. As you can see, it will take some planning to replenish your carbohydrate stores on a heavy training day.

Not only should you be concerned with the volume of carbohydrates ingested but also with the quality of ingested carbohydrates. Complex carbohydrates, such as whole grains, fruits, and vegetables, are excellent sources of carbohydrates. Refined grains, though, lose a significant amount of their nutrients during the refining process and should be avoided when possible. Limit simple carbohydrates (simple sugars), such as those found in ice cream, soda, and candy, in your diet as much as possible. Keep in mind, however, that some simple carbohydrates are good, such as those found in fruit and milk.

The glycemic index measures the effect of carbohydrate ingestion on blood glucose levels. Foods that are below 50 on the glycemic index have very little effect on blood glucose levels. However, foods that measure above 70 can cause a large increase in blood glucose levels, resulting in a significant spike in insulin (hyperinsulinemia), which in turn causes hypoglycemia (low blood sugar), and then fatigue. For this reason, it is recommended to stay away from foods that are high on the glycemic index. The one exception is during training sessions or when racing. Ingesting foods that are high on the glycemic index during a race or long training session will result in blood glucose spikes when you need them and in turn save the stored glycogen for later use.

Fats (Lipids)

Fats play many different roles in the body. They are used as a major source of energy, assist in thermoregulation, provide protection for vital organs, and assist in the transport of fat-soluble vitamins and the production of hormones. They provide a major source of energy during prolonged endurance activities below anaerobic threshold. Once ingested, fats are stored as triacylglycerol in the body and provide a large amount of energy per molecule. The average individual stores approximately 70,000 to 80,000 kCals of fats within muscle and in adipose tissue (around organs and just under the skin). This number can obviously vary from individual to individual.

There are three categories of fats: saturated fats, unsaturated fats, and trans fats. Saturated fats can be found in foods such as meats, eggs, milk, and cheese. Unsaturated fats can be either monounsaturated (found in canola oil, sunflower oil, and almonds) or polyunsaturated (found in meats, eggs, nuts, fish, fruits, and vegetables). Trans fats are found naturally in small amounts within meats and dairy products and are not of great concern. However, trans fats that are artificially made through hydrogenation are unhealthy and found in processed foods such as cakes, snacks, and fast foods.

Approximately 30 percent of your daily intake should consist of fats, with the majority coming from unsaturated fats. Less than 10 percent of your dietary intake should come from saturated fats. Stay away from trans fats, as they are detrimental to your health. Also stay away from extremely low-fat diets (<15 percent of daily intake), as they can have a strong negative impact on health and performance.

Proteins

Proteins are primarily used for anabolic processes and provide very limited energy during exercise. They are typically only relied on for energy production when glycogen stores are depleted. Proteins are vital in the recovery process as they help rebuild tissue. Excess ingested proteins are not stored in the body and are converted to either triacylglycerol or glycogen for storage. Meat, seafood, poultry, milk, cheese, eggs, and nuts are primary sources of protein in the diet.

As an athlete, you should ingest 1.2 to 2 grams of protein per kilogram of body mass each day; however, as training volume or intensity increases, you will need to increase protein ingestion to support the necessary anabolic processes that are required after training. It is important to note that taking in very large amounts of protein can place a strain on the liver and result in dehydration and electrolyte imbalance. But this is typically not a concern for healthy individuals who are not ingesting more than 4 grams per kilogram of body mass per day.

VITAMINS

Vitamins do not provide energy directly. However, they are vital in many of the chemical processes that regularly occur in the human body. Here are some common examples: B vitamins and niacin are a significant part of the chemical process that ultimately results in the production of adenosine triphosphate (ATP); vitamin D is important for bone density; and vitamin C assists in iron absorption, to name only a few.

For most healthy obstacle course racers who maintain a well-balanced diet, there is no need to supplement with vitamins. However, for those who may not be eating an adequate diet, vitamin supplementation may be beneficial.

MINERALS

Minerals are inorganic nutrients required for normal body function.

Calcium

The most abundant mineral in the human body is calcium, which plays a key role in many chemical processes in the body. Human bones consist of 60 to 70 percent calcium; therefore, it is critical for maintaining a healthy bone density.

Calcium is also stored in muscle and plays a major role in the chain of events that result in a muscle contraction. Calcium is primarily obtained by consuming dairy products.

Iron

Iron is another mineral that is necessary to maintain normal body function. It is used in the formation of hemoglobin and myoglobin. Iron is not required in large amounts and can easily be obtained through the ingestion of meat and some plant sources such as potatoes or beans. However, plants provide insufficient amounts of iron by themselves. Unless you are iron deficient or a vegetarian, there is no real need to take iron supplements. Supplementing with too much iron can also have a negative health impact.

Iron-deficient anemia results from low iron levels in the body and presents as a feeling of fatigue due to a decrease in hemoglobin. Certain populations are more prone to the development of iron-deficient anemia. Female athletes are susceptible due to iron loss occurring during the menstrual cycle, through heavy sweating during training, and through the high hemoglobin turnover rate associated with heavy training regimens. Vegetarians are also at risk due to the limited availability of iron in plants.

Phosphorus

Phosphorus is another mineral that is widely used in the body for various chemical processes. It binds with calcium to form calcium phosphate, which is vital for bone growth and development. Phosphorus is also important for protein synthesis and responsible for the formation of ATP. Phosphorus is consumed easily in most diets and can be found in meats, dairy products, and cereals.

Electrolytes

There are three minerals that are considered electrolytes: chlorine, sodium, and potassium. Electrolytes are electrically charged ions that are found within the fluids of the body. It is important to keep electrolytes balanced in the body as they help maintain homeostasis. Sodium and potassium are two electrolytes that athletes should be aware of when developing a sound nutrition plan. It is often stated that Americans ingest too much sodium within their diet, resulting in high blood pressure. While this is true, athletes should ingest greater amounts of sodium than what is recommended for the average sedentary individual, due to the excess sodium lost during training through sweat. The more you sweat, the more sodium you will lose. This is why ingestion of sodium after exercise in the heat is recommended and why many sports drinks will contain sodium. This is also why pickle juice is recommended for reducing muscle cramps in the heat. It isn't actually the "pickle" portion of the juice that is beneficial but is instead the high concentration of sodium found within pickle juice.

Potassium also helps maintain homeostasis through the electrical balance within the cells and is found in many common foods such as bananas, citrus fruits, and potatoes. A small amount of potassium is also found in fish. Individuals who maintain a healthy diet will acquire sufficient potassium without supplementation.

WATER

The human body is composed of approximately 60 to 70 percent water, which is vital for both sustaining life and for sport performance. Blood plasma in the body consists of approximately 90 percent water and is responsible for the transportation of gasses, nutrients, and other compounds throughout the body. As water is an excellent conductor of heat, blood plasma is also responsible for thermoregulation. Because water levels are vital to the body, when exercising it is important to develop and maintain a sound hydration plan.

During exercise water is lost through sweating and through respiration. As you sweat, water moves from the interstitial space and exits the body through eccrine sweat glands in order to evaporate on the skin and cool the body. Water from plasma will move from the blood vessels into the interstitial space to replace the lost water and equalize pressure between the blood vessels and interstitial space. This action results in an overall decrease in plasma volume and a decreased ability to cool the body. Water loss during exercise can negatively impact both performance and health. Water loss that is equivalent to approximately a 2 percent decrease in body mass will negatively impact performance. As the water loss reaches a 5 percent decrease in body mass, there will be a negative impact on overall health. One of the primary health concerns with dehydration is the inability to properly thermoregulate, leading to heat-related illnesses.

Because of the high volume of fluid lost during prolonged exercise, the recommendations for daily water intake for average individuals (1.5 to 3 liters/day) cannot be applied to obstacle course racing. Due to this fact, it is important to replace fluid that is lost during training or competition.

One of the best methods for determining water loss is to weigh yourself both before and after your training session. It is important to weigh unclothed before and after so that you are not measuring the volume of water retained in your clothes after training. The difference in weight between the before and after measures represents the volume of fluid lost during the session. The next step is to replace each pound lost with approximately 24 ounces of fluid. This rehydration recommendation assumes that you were properly hydrated prior to the exercise bout.

NUTRITION AND EXERCISE

To promote recovery, positive adaptations, and increased performance, spend some time developing a sound nutritional strategy. There are four basic areas to consider when developing a nutrition plan for exercise. The first is the type of nutrition, carbohydrates, lipids, proteins, etc., you will ingest. The second involves the quality of nutrition: choose high-quality foods. The third involves the volume, or caloric intake, of your nutrition plan; and the fourth consideration deals with the timing of the meals.

Before Training or Racing

When examining prerace/pretraining nutrition, the timing, quantity, and type of nutrition must be addressed. Meals should be eaten two to four hours prior to competition. Eat light foods that will provide energy but that do not take a prolonged time to digest. For example, slow-cooked oatmeal, bagels, or fruits make an excellent breakfast, but stay away from the sausage, egg, and cheese sandwich.

Training or racing without eating prior can negatively impact performance and possibly health, especially on high-intensity days. Not eating prior to a workout can lead to low blood glucose levels, resulting in feelings of fatigue and dizziness. There will be a larger effect at higher intensities due to an increased reliance on glycogen and glucose as primary energy sources. At race pace during a 10km obstacle course race, you will utilize 100 percent of your glucose and glycogen as a fuel source. Low blood glucose levels occur most commonly in individuals who skip breakfast for their morning training.

It is also not recommended to eat a large meal just prior to a training bout or race as it will often leave you feeling sluggish and with gastrointestinal distress. During exercise, blood flow will be directed to areas that need it most, such as the working muscles and the skin for cooling. It will also be redirected from areas that need it the least, such as the digestive tract. After eating a meal, blood is redirected to the digestive tract in order to properly digest the food. So, if a meal is eaten prior to exercise, these two systems are at odds. During exercise, inadequate blood flow will be redirected to the digestive system in an attempt to properly digest a meal, leading to gastrointestinal distress.

In general, it is recommended to avoid most foods that are high on the glycemic index. However, ingesting carbohydrates that are high on the index prior to the start of exercise will help spare glycogen during an endurance event lasting longer than an hour. Carbohydrates high on the glycemic index will increase blood glucose levels fairly quickly, which in turn will spare glycogen stored in the liver. Carbohydrates, such as sports gels, can be ingested approximately 5 to 10 minutes prior to the start of exercise. Supplementing with carbohydrates is only recommended for exercise lasting longer than an hour. Do not ingest sports gels more than 10 minutes prior to the start of the event, as this could cause an early blood glucose spike, leading to an overshoot of insulin, low blood sugar levels, and fatigue.

During an Event

During training sessions and races that last longer than an hour, you will need to take in carbohydrates. Glycogen stores are topped off at around 2,000 to 2,500 kCals in the human body and therefore become a limiting factor for energy production through oxidative processes during prolonged exercise. As mentioned, ingesting carbohydrates increases blood glucose levels and therefore spares glycogen stores in the liver, offsetting glycogen depletion and the resulting fatigue. Keep in mind that glycogen is utilized at a much faster rate during high-intensity exercise.

When training or racing at high intensity for longer than an hour, you should ingest 30 to 60 grams of carbohydrates every 45 to 60 minutes of exercise. This is also true for sessions occurring at lower intensities that last longer than 90 minutes. Choose carbohydrates that are easily digested and high on the glycemic index to enter the system quickly. Energy gels and sports drinks are typical choices. In comparison, sports bars enter the system at a slower rate.

When choosing what food source to use during training and racing, there are important aspects to consider. First, what is in the supplement? The nutrition label located on the package tells you how many carbohydrates are contained inside and what other supplements it may provide (protein, caffeine, etc.) as well. Another consideration is taste, which is especially true of sports drinks. If you do not like the taste, you will consume the substance less often, which will destroy your nutritional plan for that race. The last thing to consider is how your body reacts to the supplement. It is important to know how your body responds to a specific gel, bar, or drink, because the last thing you want to have to deal with is gastrointestinal distress during the race. Always try a new product on a training day prior to using it in a race.

It is vital to remain hydrated when training and racing. This rule is even more critical on hot and humid days as you will lose a greater amount of fluid on those days. As mentioned, dehydration results in a decrease in performance and leads to heat-related illnesses. You can hydrate with water, sports drinks, or a combination of both. Hydrating with water during sessions lasting less than an hour and a half will be sufficient in most cases. High-intensity activities lasting an hour and a half could benefit from supplementing fluid intake with a sports drink. However, in activities lasting longer than an hour and a half, it would be beneficial to use a sports drink to provide hydration, electrolyte replacement, and carbohydrates.

It is impossible to completely maintain hydration levels during a long training session or race in the heat, resulting in dehydration. Therefore, it is vital that you develop a hydration plan and stick with it throughout the session. Thirst is a mechanism that lets us know that dehydration is setting in and that we need to drink. During exercise, if you wait until you are thirsty to drink, it is already too late and you have already begun a downward spiral that can lead to decreased performance and the development of a heat-related illness.

Wearing a hydration pack when running trails is a great way to stay hydrated. Hydration packs allow you to carry a large volume of water without difficulty and to drink easier and more often when running trails. While a hydration pack is ideal for training, it may not be ideal for a race as you must carry that extra weight on every obstacle.

Hyponatremia, a fluid–electrolyte imbalance, is not typical in shorter races and is much more common in ultra-endurance events. So, unless you are competing in an ultra-distance race, hyponatremia most likely will not be a concern. Hyponatremia occurs when electrolyte levels are extremely low, affecting the ratio of fluid and electrolytes. The imbalance created by a high concentration of water and low concentration of sodium can result in the following: headache, nausea, cramping, seizures, coma, heart attack, and death. Hyponatremia occurs during prolonged events where the athletes ingest large volumes of fluid without replenishing lost electrolytes, resulting in an electrolyte imbalance. Taking in electrolytes during prolonged exercise will help offset this imbalance.

After Training and Competition

Recovery is an important component of any training program, and nutrition is key in the recovery process. What you ingest after a workout is just as important as what you take in before and during a workout. Training applies the necessary stress for positive adaptations and eventual performance increases to occur. However, this stress results in catabolic responses during exercise. It is the anabolic process, which occurs after exercise, that ultimately results in improved performance. Post-exercise recovery not only helps with the anabolic processes but also begins the refueling process.

You must start refueling within one to two hours after completion of exercise. The typical recommendation to optimize recovery is within 45 to 60 minutes. The four primary nutrients to ingest are water, electrolytes, carbohydrates, and proteins. Replace each pound of fluid lost through sweating with approximately 24 ounces of fluid. Use of a sports drink can be beneficial for both fluid and electrolyte replacement.

Carbohydrates and proteins should be ingested using a 4:1 ratio (4 grams of carbohydrates to 1 gram of proteins). Carbohydrates are necessary for replenishing glycogen stores, and proteins are vital for supporting the anabolic processes after exercise. You cannot completely replenish glycogen stores directly after a workout; it will be an ongoing process throughout the rest of the day. Ingesting protein after exercise also assists in glucose and amino acid uptake into the muscles as well as influencing insulin levels. These factors are why the 4:1 ratio has been so successful during the recovery process. Recovery sports drink mixes that provide the necessary 4:1 ratio have been shown to be very effective at aiding recovery. Research has demonstrated that chocolate milk provides the same ratio and the same benefits.

BODY COMPOSITION

Body composition is the composition of the body in relation to fat and fat-free mass (muscle, bone, tissue, etc.). One of the most accurate and most commonly used methods for determining body composition is body fat percentage, which examines the percentage of fat to fat-free mass. For example, a body fat recording of 15 percent indicates that the individual's body mass is 15 percent fat and 85 percent fat-free mass. Monitoring body fat percentage is an excellent way to track changes in your body composition.

For General Health

Many people begin obstacle course racing for health reasons and the desire to get into better shape. Currently in America, more than 65 percent of people are classified as overweight and more than 30 percent are classified as obese. Being overweight or obese can result in various negative health conditions such as hypertension, high cholesterol (LDL) levels, type II diabetes, cardiovascular disease, certain types of cancer, gall bladder disease, joint problems, breathing problems, and all-cause mortality. Keep in mind that overweight individuals who are physically active are less likely to develop cardiovascular disease than individuals who are thin but sedentary.

If you are participating in OCR for health reasons or because you enjoy the activity, you need not worry too much about body composition. By training and eating right, body composition will take care of itself over time. The recommended body fat percentage range is 8 to 19 percent for males and 17 to 28 percent for females. Maintaining a healthy body composition within these recommended ranges is ideal for promoting optimal health. Classification of overweight begins at a body fat percentage greater than 20 percent for men and 30 percent for women. As body fat percentage increases beyond the initial classification of overweight, health risk increases significantly. Remember, though, that having too little body fat can also have a negative impact on health. The essential body fat percentage for normal bodily functions is 4 percent for males and 12 percent for females.

For Competition

If you wish to truly compete in obstacle course racing, you will need to be a little more concerned with body composition. Overall body mass, regardless of body composition, affects OCR performance. The greater your body mass, the harder it will be to perform many of the obstacles required in OCR as most require you to move your body mass during climbing and overhead obstacles. As an athlete you do not want to decrease your overall mass by decreasing lean muscle mass. Instead, you want to decrease overall mass by decreasing body fat.

The recommended ranges for body compositions for competitive obstacle course racers are 4 to 10 percent for males and 12 to 20 percent for females. While a low body fat percentage may be desirable for competition, there are a few factors you must consider. The first is that a low body fat composition is very difficult to achieve and maintain. The closer an athlete gets to the lower end of the recommended athletic range, the greater the risk of decreased performance and compromised health. The second consideration is that not everyone will respond in the same manner to decreased body fat percentages. I have worked with elite-level athletes whose performance dropped when their body fat percent became too low, even though it was above the recommendations for an elite-level racer. When or if your body fat percentage drops into the lower range, make sure that you carefully monitor both performance and health. The goal is to be as light as possible without negatively impacting health or performance.

Measuring Body Composition

If you are serious about performance, you will want to track changes in body composition over time. Different methods for determining body composition are described in this section, along with the advantages and disadvantages of each. Choose a method that is both accurate and feasible.

Body Mass Index

Body mass index (BMI) is solely based on height and weight. It provides a simple and easy way to determine if an individual is underweight, normal, over-weight, or obese and can be calculated using either the metric or the English/imperial system. Formulas for both systems have been provided below. Once you calculate your BMI, you can then refer to the following chart to determine which category you fall into:

English $\quad$ $BMI = 703 \times weight\ (lb) \div height^2\ (inches^2)$

Metric $\quad$ $BMI = weight\ (kg) \div height^2\ (M^2)$

If your BMI is <18.5, you are considered underweight; normal BMI falls between 18.5 and 24.9; overweight is considered to be between 25 and 29.9; and obese is classified as a BMI ≥ 30.

Body mass index is an excellent tool for estimating body composition for large-scale populations, but it loses validity when examining individual athletes. The reason for this is the fact that muscle is denser than fat and therefore weighs more. At the time of this writing, I weigh 194 pounds and my height is 71.75 inches. This would make my BMI 26.49, classifying me as overweight. However, my body fat is at 8 percent, and therefore I am not overweight. This demonstrates the primary disadvantage of relying on BMI to determine body composition when working with athletes.

Bioelectrical Impedance

Bioelectrical impedance systems use electrical currents in order to estimate body fat percentage. These systems require contact with either the hands or the feet. Once contact is made, the system passes an electrical current through the body to measure resistance to flow. Lean body tissue contains high concentrations of water, and therefore the electrical current passes through the body easily. Fat contains little water and therefore provides resistance to flow. As fat stores increase, resistance to flow also increases. It is a fast and easy method for determining body composition. However, bioelectrical impedance systems are neither reliable nor accurate.

Bioelectrical impedance systems rely heavily on the ability of the electrical current to easily flow through water, therefore hydration levels significantly impact body fat percentage estimates. Your hydration levels during training will continuously fluctuate, especially in the hotter months, resulting in large fluctuations of bioelectrical impedance readings. Due to the large fluctuations in hydration levels and the inherent variability in these machines, I do not recommend them for measuring body composition.

Hydrostatic Weighing

Hydrostatic weighing (underwater weighing) has long been considered the gold standard for determining body composition. This method is based on Archimedes' principle, which states that the weight of water displaced by the body is equivalent to the buoyant forces acting on that body. Lean body mass (muscles, bones, organs, etc.) has greater density than water and therefore sinks, and fat is less dense than water and therefore floats. The amount of lean mass and fat mass will determine how buoyant an individual is in water.

While hydrostatic weighing is considered the gold standard, the process requires large specialized equipment and trained professionals. This method involves the use of a water tank large enough for a human to completely submerge under water without touching the sides or bottom of the tank. The athlete must also be physically able to completely submerge, exhale as much air as possible, and remain still long enough to obtain a steady measure of underwater weight. This process makes it difficult for those who are uncomfortable underwater.

Dual-Energy X-Ray Absorptiometry

Dual-energy X-ray absorptiometry (DXA) determines body composition through the use of two low energy X-ray beams and has the ability to accurately measure density and distinguish between fat and fat-free mass. Due to this method's accuracy and reliability, it is now often considered the best way to determine body composition. However, the DXA system is extremely expensive and requires very specialized skill to operate.

Calipers

More than any of the methods previously mentioned, I recommend the use of skin-fold calipers for determining body composition. Skin-fold calipers are accurate, inexpensive, easy to use, and far more accessible and affordable than the other methods. Skin-fold calipers work by pinching a fold of skin and fat and measuring the thickness of the fold. From the skin-fold measurements, total fat stores are estimated using simple formulas. Skin-fold calipers cost anywhere from $25 to $200. The major differences between a lower- and higher-cost caliper are accuracy and durability.

Conducting skin-fold testing is relatively simple but does take some practice to master. There are different tests used to measure skin folds, but the three-site test is the most widely used. The most common body sites used for men are the chest, abdomen, and thigh. The three most common sites for females are the triceps, iliac, and thigh.

When conducting skin-fold measures, it is important to accurately measure each site as described: Position the hand so that the fingers point down, and fold the skin between the thumb and index finger as shown in figure 5.1. Once your fingers are positioned over the correct spot, pinch the skin, bringing it up into a fold. For an accurate measurement, pinch skin and fat only. Too large a pinch typically results in getting muscle, which results in an inaccurate measurement. Next, place the caliper pincers directly below your thumb and index finger with the gauge facing up so that you can read it. Once the caliper is in position, allow the calipers to close on the fold by slowly releasing the lever. Do not release the skin fold with your fingers until you record the measurement and remove the calipers. If you release the skin fold prior to the calipers, it can be slightly painful. Take three to four measurements at each site to ensure consistent readings. It is important to measure precisely where described in order to obtain valid measurements. It is also important to be consistent with your measurements. The following instructions will provide you the necessary information to conduct a simple three-site test.

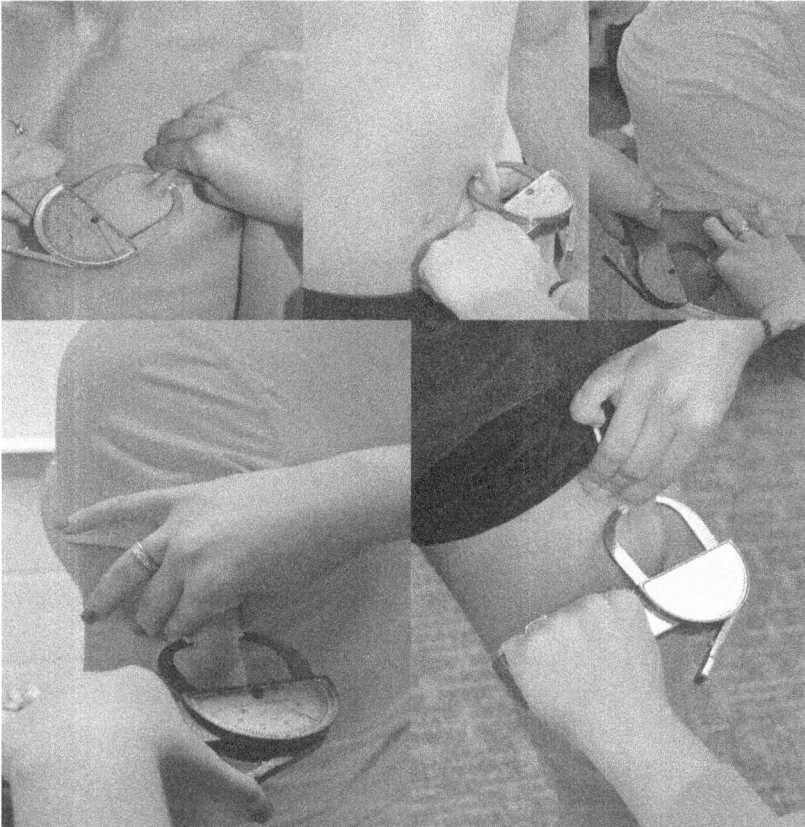

Figure 5.1. Skin folds. *Will Peveler.*

Chest. The chest site is located along the outer edge of the pectoralis major at the midpoint of the muscle. The skin fold should be in line with the outer edge of the muscle, as shown in fig. 5.1.

Abdomen. The abdomen site is located in line with the navel and one inch toward the side. Fold the skin vertically, not horizontally.

Iliac. The iliac site is located just above the hip bone. Fold the skin in line with the natural crease at the hip bone.

Triceps. The triceps sites are located at the back of the arm, centered and halfway between the shoulder and elbow. Fold the skin vertically.

Thigh. The thigh site for this test is located on the center line of the thigh halfway between the hip and the patella. Fold the skin vertically. When working with athletic women, it can be difficult to properly obtain the correct measurements. As the thigh is a primary storage location for fat in women and athletic women have significant muscle mass in the legs, it may take a little harder pinch in order to accurately measure.

Once you have recorded all three sites, take the sum of the readings and plug the necessary data into the necessary equations. For men:

Body Density = 1.10938 – (.0008267 × sum of skin folds) + (.0000016 × [sum of skin folds]^2) – (.0002574 × age)

And for women:

Body Density = 1.0994921 – (.0009929 × sum of skin folds) + (.0000023 × [sum of skin folds]^2) – (.0001392 × age)

This first step gives you the estimated body density for the three-site skin-fold test. Once body density has been established, the next step is to determine body fat percentage using the following formula:

Body Fat% = (4.95 ÷ Body Density) – 4.50 × 100

Example equation:

Male: Age = 25; Chest = 5, Abdominal = 9, Thigh = 4 (Total = 18)
Body Density = 1.10938 – (.0008267 × 18) + (.0000016 × [18]^2) – (.0002574 × 25)
BD = 1.088
Body Fat% = (4.95 ÷1.088) – 4.50 × 100 = 4.96 percent

WEIGHT MANAGEMENT

Whether your weight management goal is for weight loss, health, or competition, there are a few important concepts to keep in mind. The first and foremost is patience. No one puts on excess weight overnight, and therefore it is unrealistic to believe that you can lose it overnight. Remain patient, avoid undue frustration, and stick with the plan. It is very common to become frustrated with your progression. When things get frustrating, ask yourself: Do I want to be standing here a year from now having lost weight, or do I want to be standing here a year from now saying I wish I would have stuck with it and lost weight? An important tool to help eliminate frustration is tracking your weight loss over time. It is important to note that weight fluctuates from day to day. Do not let this phenomenon discourage you from your ultimate goal.

Second, recognize that weight loss is not an easy process. You must be prepared for hard, physical work in order to achieve your goal. Additionally, you will need to implement a safe and healthy diet to accomplish your goal. Ignoring these simple facts will result in frustration and failure.

Finally, it is important to understand that not everyone responds to weight loss in the same manner. Do not compare your weight loss to another's. This is unrealistic and counterproductive. However, it does not mean that you cannot work in a group toward the same goal. As a matter of fact, working with a support group can be very beneficial. Just do not compare your journey with other members of the group.

Factors that Affect Weight Management

Genetics

Genetics plays a major role when it comes to body composition. Research shows that children of overweight parents are much more likely to be overweight than children of non-overweight parents. How body fat is distributed in the body is also strongly affected by genetics. It is easier for some people to lose weight while others continuously struggle. However, this does not mean that you are fated to be overweight just because you have a genetic predisposition toward weight gain. All it means is that you need to be more careful of how you eat and that you need to exercise on a regular basis.

Lifestyle

While genetics is one of the key factors in determining body composition, it is lifestyle choices that have the greatest effect on body composition. Lifestyle is defined as the daily choices you make that affect how you live your life. The two key lifestyle choices that affect body composition are physical activity and diet.

Eating out often is one of the common mistakes people make. Food offered at sit-down and fast-food restaurants typically provides more calories in one meal than most people need in one day. At this point, I am only focusing on the caloric content and not the nutritional value of the food. Also, keep in mind that this is a generic statement that covers the vast majority of restaurants and that there are restaurants that provide good portion sizes and healthy options.

It would be unrealistic to never eat out or grab something from a fast-food restaurant. Here are a few guidelines that can help you when you do choose to eat out. The first recommendation requires a little planning on your part. Determine the caloric content of the foods that are offered at the restaurant you plan to visit. Many restaurants provide this information on their online menu.

Another option is to decrease your portion size. Many restaurants will have different options when it comes to portion size, which allows you to order the portion size that best suits your needs. If there is only one option for portion size and it is too large for you, simply do not eat it all. Just because you order the meal does not mean that you have to eat all of it in one sitting. Too often I have ordered a meal, eaten the entire thing, and then felt miserable afterward. One way to avoid this scenario is to portion your meal when you receive it, only eat the prescribed portion, and take the rest home for another meal. If you do not have the willpower to stop eating when you are full, then ask for a "to go" box at the beginning of the meal and place the portion that you do not plan to eat in the box to take home. One of my favorite places to eat has a very large seafood pasta that I love. I can easily split it into three meals. If you are eating with someone who has similar taste, you can also consider sharing a meal.

Preparing and eating meals at home, if done correctly, is the best option when it comes to managing body composition. Ideally, you want to prepare meals from fresh foods that are not excessively processed. Eating healthy at home is not as expensive as one might think, and you will discover that it is much less expensive than eating out. Another misconception is that you have to spend hours in the kitchen in order to cook healthy meals. While the time to cook a meal does vary, depending on what you are cooking, there are many healthy meals that can be prepared quickly. If you are not familiar with healthy cooking, consider buying a cookbook that focuses on the subject. You will soon find healthy, tasty meals that are easy to prepare.

Even when eating healthy at home, be aware of portion sizes. Modern dish-ware has gotten larger over time, and if you fill your plate you will probably take in more calories than you need. Most of us were raised on "cleaning" our plate before leaving the table in order not to waste food. While the logic behind this practice is understandable, it is much better to listen to your stomach and stop eating when you are full.

Meal planning is one method that will save you time and effort and allow for healthy meals. The first step to eating healthy begins when you make your grocery list. Making a healthy grocery list and sticking to that list will help eliminate unhealthy eating, and prevent those impulse buys when you walk past an item that looks appetizing. If you do not buy junk food, you can't eat junk food. It is also not a good idea to grocery shop after a hard workout when you are tired and hungry. Whenever I shop when I am hungry, my grocery basket always seems to be fuller and filled with some less-than-healthy choices.

Always read the nutrition label when purchasing foods in order to determine amounts of cholesterol, sodium, sugar, calories, etc. When examining the caloric content, it is important to determine how many calories per serving as well as serving size. For example, a serving size may be a half cup and a caloric content of 80 calories per serving. But if you ingest a full cup, then the caloric content would be 160 calories.

Another valuable tool for weight management is a nutritional log. Keeping a nutritional log of everything you eat for the day will allow you to determine the volume of calories consumed. This is an eye opener for many individuals who do not realize how many calories they ingest in a single day, and can be a very effective tool for demonstrating the need for a lifestyle change. When keeping a nutritional log, record everything that you ingest and the calorie content of each. Keep in mind this includes everything you eat, including snacks, and everything you drink. Keeping a nutrition log is tedious work and may not be something that you want to maintain on a permanent basis, but try to keep a log until you have made the proper adjustments to your eating habits.

Goals for Weight Management

Setting goals for your weight management program is an important part of the process of losing weight. Weight loss will be challenging for everyone, and therefore it is important to set realistic long- and short-term goals. Setting a weight-loss goal of 10 pounds over an 8- to 10-week period would be realistic for most individuals, whereas setting a goal of losing 10 pounds in a week would be very unrealistic. Setting unrealistic goals will negatively impact your weight-management program and lead to serious discouragement. As mentioned previously, losing weight takes a long period of time and you must remain patient. Setting short-term goals in conjunction with your long-term goal will allow you to monitor small steps in progression over time and help limit discouragement.

Safe, effective, and sustainable weight loss is considered to be roughly a loss of one pound per week. There will be weeks when you lose more and others when you lose less. Understand that weight will fluctuate, and do not become discouraged.

In order to optimally set weight-management goals, know what your current body composition is as well as your desired body composition. The first step in this process is to determine your current body weight and body fat percentage, discussed previously in this chapter. The next step is to determine your desired body composition. While elite-level OCR athletes have very low body fat percentages (males as low as 4 percent and females as low as 11 percent), this is an unrealistic goal for many. Typically, the goal of 8 to 19 percent for males and 17 to 28 percent for females is a good and achievable goal. I understand that I have provided a wide range of body fat percentages for both male and female racers. However, where you would like to be in that range is a personal choice. Once you have determined your current weight, current body fat percentage, and desired body fat percentage, use the formulas below to determine weight loss.

(Current Weight) × (Current Body Fat Percentage) = Weight of Fat in the Body
Current Weight – Weight of Fat in the Body = Weight of Fat Free Mass
1 – Desired Body Fat Percentage = Percent Fat-Free Mass
Weight of Fat-Free Mass ÷ Percent Fat-Free Mass = Desired Body Weight
Current Body Weight – Desired Body Weight = Desired Weight Loss

Example equation:

Male: 210 lbs: Currently 22% Body Fat; Desires 12% Body Fat
(210 lbs) × (.22) = 46.2 lbs
210 lbs – 46.2 lbs = 163.8 lbs
1 – .12 = .88
163.8 lbs ÷ .88 = 186.14 lbs
210 lbs – 186.14 lbs = 23.86 lbs

In the example above, a 210-pound male with a body fat percentage of 22 was able to determine that his desired body weight would be 186.14 pounds and that he would need to lose 23.86 pounds to reach the goal of 10 percent body fat. Remember, the goal is really about body composition and not weight. Because muscle is denser than fat, it weighs more. As you train and improve, muscle will hypertrophy over time and increase the weight of your lean body mass. Therefore, you will need to periodically rework the equations and adjust your weight-management goals.

Caloric Balance

In its most simplistic form, weight management is all about caloric balance. When your caloric consumption is equivalent to your caloric expenditure, your body composition will remain at a near constant. If you consume more calories than you expend, you will gain weight. If you consume less calories than you expend, then weight will decrease over time. It would be extremely difficult to count the precise number of calories consumed and expended during a single day. However, counting calories in and calories out as precisely as possible will give you a good starting point. Some days you will take in slightly more than you use and others you will take in slightly less than you use. However, an overall deficit will balance out over time, resulting in weight loss. Keep in mind that if caloric intake remains too low for too long, metabolism can decrease, which is counterproductive to weight management. Extremely low caloric intake can also lead to catabolism of lean tissue, primarily muscle, in the body, which is also counterproductive.

It is commonly recommended that males consume between 2,000 and 2,500 calories per day and that females take in between 1,500 to 1,800 calories per day. It is important to keep in mind that these recommendations are for the average male and female who do not participate in regular exercise, and therefore would represent insufficient calories for most racers. A long obstacle course race can burn more calories than the average recommended calories per day. In order to optimally determine caloric requirements, you must first estimate how much you utilize on any given day.

The first step in determining caloric balance is to measure basal metabolic rate (BMR) or resting metabolic rate (RMR), which is the minimum energy required to properly maintain normal body function at rest. Both BMR and RMR will provide similar numbers, but differ in methodology of measurement. Resting metabolic rate typically provides numbers that are slightly higher than BMR, but the terms are often used interchangeably. For the purpose of this book and to eliminate confusion, I will use the term "basal metabolic rate." Basal metabolic rate generally ranges from around 1,100 kCals to 2,100 kCals per day. It is the minimum energy required just to exist, and any physical activity conducted throughout the day will add to basal metabolic rate. This is why the typical daily caloric recommendations for individuals range from 1,600 kCals/day for females to 2,500 kCals/day for males. These numbers go up for physically active males and females.

A linear relationship exists between heart rate and increased metabolism (typically estimated by VO^2), and therefore heart rate can be used to estimate basal metabolic rate. In order to estimate BMR using heart rate, you will need a heart rate monitor that estimates kCals at rest. Record caloric expenditure at rest for 10 minutes and multiply by 6 to determine caloric expenditure for an hour. The resultant number is then multiplied by 24 to determine caloric expenditure for an entire day (BMR).

Laboratory testing for BMR and RMR is time consuming and expensive. Therefore, formulas are often used to estimate both. While formulas are not as accurate as direct measures, they can provide a fairly accurate estimation and a great place to begin. The following formula is used for men:

$$\text{kCals/day} = 66 + (13.7 \times \text{body weight in kg}) + (5 \times \text{height in cm}) - (6.9 \times \text{age})$$

and this one is for women:

$$\text{kCals/day} = 665 + (9.6 \times \text{body weight in kg}) + (1.7 \times \text{height in cm}) - (4.7 \times \text{age})$$

Here is an example equation for a man, 180 lbs (81.63 kg), 72 in tall (182.88 cm), age 25:

$$\text{kCals/day} = 66 + (13.7 \times 81.63) + (5 \times 182.88) - (6.9 \times 25) = 1,926.23 \text{ kCals}$$

After basal metabolic rate has been determined, add caloric expenditure due to activity to the equation. If you had a morning run that used 600 kCals, then went for a short hike with your kids and used 200 kCals, you would then add those 800 kCals to your basal metabolic rate. Any physical activity (mowing the lawn, cleaning the house, etc.) above resting needs to be added to BMR. Keep in mind that this methodology is not 100 percent accurate and only gives you a ballpark number. This is why counting calories ingested, counting calories utilized, and measuring changes in body mass are all important components of weight management. If you lose or gain too much weight, adjust caloric intake accordingly.

Most heart rate monitors can estimate energy expenditure for endurance activities based on heart rate. The estimations provided by most heart rate monitors will be decently accurate for endurance activities. However, heart rate monitors cannot provide an accurate estimation of caloric expenditure for activities such as interval training or resistance training. For these activities you can use metabolic equivalents (METs) to help you determine energy expenditure for your specific activities. One MET is equal to 3.5 ml/kg/min, which represents a resting state. So, each MET you go above 1 is an activity level above your resting state.

The first thing to determine when using METs to calculate energy expenditure is the particular METs for the activity that you are conducting. If you are lifting weights, the METs will range from 3 (very light) to 6 (vigorous).

Determine where your overall intensity was for that session. An example of a 3 would be when you first start lifting and you are working on technique, not pushing a lot of weight and stopping at a set number of reps before volitional exhaustion. An example of a 6 would be when you are lifting at high intensity to volitional exhaustion with every set. Muscular endurance activities will fall somewhere between 8 and 10 METs. Push-ups until volitional exhaustion for each set would be an example of an 8, and burpees until volitional exhaustion for each set would be an example of a 10. You can also use METs to estimate energy expenditure for endurance activities as well. And you can find the METs for running at any given speed. For example, the METs for running at a 12-minute-per-mile pace would be about 8, and a 6-minute-per-mile pace would be about 15. Be careful when using METs based on minute-per-mile pace, however, as you could be running an average 10-minute-per-mile pace simply because you are running a very hilly course. Your speed of running will not always measure intensity or energy expenditure.

To calculate energy expenditure from METs, you will need your current body mass in kilograms for the equation I provide below, the time spent conducting the activity, and the METs for that activity. When looking at time for running, it is fairly simple: know your start and stop times. When looking at something such as a resistance training session, however, it is not as straightforward. If you conduct your resistance training and stay on task, you can count your entire session as time. However, if you spend a lot of time talking and extend an hour session into an hour and a half, then you only count the hour. Keep in mind that these are estimations, but you want to be as accurate as possible. Following is the formula:

(METs)(Body mass in kilograms)/60 = kCals/min

And here is an example problem for an 81.63-kg male athlete conducting resistance training for 45 minutes at a vigorous intensity:

(6 METs)(81.63 kg)/60 = 8.16 kCals/min
(8.16 kCals/min)(45 min) = 367.2 kCals

As you can see in the example above, this individual's caloric expenditure would be 367.2 kCals for that particular workout. I used the same numbers from the previous example where I calculated basal metabolic rate. So, at this point in the day this individual would have expended 2,293.43 kCals (BMR of 1,926.23 kCals + resistance training of 367.2 kCals). You would add in any other significant energy expenditure throughout the day to get a total for the day. You would then subtract energy consumed during the day to determine your net caloric balance.

When training for OCR, make sure to replenish the calories used throughout the day. This process is vital for energy replenishment as well as for driving anabolic processes for recovery. As mentioned previously, it is all about manipulating caloric balance in order to reach your specific weight-management goals. If you know how many calories you burned throughout the day, you know how many you need to replace. This is where your nutrition log can be helpful. By reading the caloric content of the food you consume and keeping track of the totals, you can compare caloric expenditure to caloric intake. Keep in mind that it is not just about the volume of nutrients but the quality of the nutrients as well.

Fad Diets

One of the biggest mistakes that people make in the pursuit of their desired body mass is looking for shortcuts. Unfortunately, there are no safe or sustainable shortcuts to weight management. This tendency for individuals to look for the fastest and easiest way to lose weight has resulted in a market for fad diets. There is no short, fast, easy, or magical way to weight loss. It is a long and gradual process that requires dedication and work. Stay away from fad diets—they do not work. When it comes to weight loss, if it sounds too good to be true, then it is. Fad diet programs result in no change in body composition at best and lead to health-related problems at worst.

In recent history, low-carbohydrate and no-carbohydrate diets have been pushed as a healthy and fast way to lose weight. However, there is nothing healthy about a low-carb or no-carb diet. This is doubly true for an endurance athlete. There are three primary reasons to stay away from a low-carb diet. The first and foremost is that the only source of fuel that the central nervous system and the brain can use is glycogen (the storage form of carbohydrates). Inadequate supplies of glycogen result in mental confusion and fatigue. As a survival mechanism, the body will produce glycogen by breaking down protein in the body. Excess protein is not stored in the body, and therefore muscle is degraded in order to provide the protein required for conversion to glycogen.

Use of lipids as a fuel will also be compromised due to low glycogen stores. As stated previously, lipids require glycogen in order to be completely catabolized for energy. Low glycogen stores and compromised lipid catabolism results in a decrease in pH (i.e., increased acidity). Other common complications of a low-carb diet are dehydration, electrolyte imbalance, strain on the liver, and strain on the kidneys.

A low-carbohydrate diet will negatively impact OCR training and performance. Glycogen stores are extremely important when training or racing at high intensities. Because glycogen stores are limited to around 2,000 kCals, you do not want to begin a training session or race with low glycogen stores. You will fatigue early and to a greater extent, and you will have trouble thinking clearly.

It would be untrue to state that you cannot lose weight through a low-carbohydrate diet. However, the weight that is lost is not entirely due to decreased lipid stores and instead will be a result of significant lean tissue loss, water loss, and lipid loss. Loss of muscle mass will have a strong negative impact on sport performance. There is also no need to take in excess carbohydrates, as excess carbohydrates will be converted to and stored as lipids.

Another commonly used fad diet for weight management is the use of diet pills. Diet pills are considered a supplement and therefore fall outside FDA regulations on foods. This allows companies to make blatantly false claims without fear of prosecution. The combination of no FDA oversight and people being desperate to lose weight has resulted in the development of a multibillion-dollar diet pill industry. Over the counter diet pills do not work as advertised and can lead to health complications.

Because of this risk, it is not recommended to use diet pills as a source of weight management. Not all, but most diet pills contain stimulants that increase metabolism, which in turn greatly increases resting heart rate and can cause heart palpitations and other medical complications. Because exercise naturally increases heart rate, diet pills can elevate that increase. On hot, humid days when blood plasma volume drops significantly due to sweating, the use of diet pills can apply excess strain on the heart.

It would be impractical to list and discuss all the fad diets that are currently being pushed, and therefore I will just give you some basic advice here. First, as mentioned previously, if it sounds too good to be true, then it most likely is. Weight loss requires time and effort, and there is no substitute. Weight management requires that you increase caloric expenditure through physical activity and that you eat a well-balanced diet that meets all your nutritional needs.

And second, you cannot "target" fat. Fat is fat, and there is no "special" type of fat in the body. Nor can you "target" specific storage locations of fat. There is not a special exercise or diet that will target belly or hip fat. With increases in physical activity, you will see an increase in fat stored in muscle, needed for increased energy availability during exercise, and a decrease in adipose storage.

ERGOGENIC AIDS

The word "ergogenic" means work enhancing. In the arena of sports performance, ergogenic aids are any aids that increase performance. Ergogenic aids
do this in three basic ways. The first is that they directly increase performance
during an event. The second is that they promote recovery between bouts.
And third, they allow for better training in order to improve later performance.
When considering ergogenic aids, it is important to examine their effectiveness,
known and possible side effects, ethics, and legality.

Ethics, Legality, and Regulations

Athletes are very focused on finding ways to improve performance, and
ergogenic aids can provide a pathway for such improvement. However, when
choosing ergogenic aids, the legality and ethics of specific ergogenic aids
must be considered. Ethics can be very subjective and are typically based on
an individual's morals and sense of right and wrong. What one person may
see as ethical, others may not. However, there is no such gray area when
looking at rules and laws. Every sport has a set of rules that competitors must
adhere to in order to compete. The United States Anti-Doping Agency has
a list of banned substances that they test for, which is discussed in greater
detail below. There are also laws that prohibit certain substances, such as
steroids.

In sports there is a basic premise that all competition is conducted on an even
playing field and that there are no unfair advantages. Any differences in performance should be based strictly on genetics, training, tactics, and ergogenic aids
that are permitted by the sport's governing body. If an ergogenic aid is illegal,
such as steroids, then it is also against regulations and hopefully counter to the
established ethical guidelines of the athlete.

Many of the obstacle course race series have signed on to the United States
Anti-Doping Agency (USADA), which is under the World Anti-Doping Agency
(WADA). The International Olympic Committee created WADA in order to
regulate the use of ergogenic aids in sports. The charge of this committee is to
create a list of banned substances, develop rules, test for banned substances, and
enforce rules. The United States Anti-Doping Agency has joined WADA and is
responsible for implementing WADA regulations in the United States.

When determining whether a substance should be banned or not, WADA
examines three main areas during deliberation:

1. Is the substance illegal?
2. Does the substance pose a serious health risk?
3. Does the substance give the athlete an unfair advantage over their competitors?

An answer of yes to one or more of these questions can result in the substance being placed on the banned-substance list.

You are ultimately responsible for knowing what is on the banned-substance list and ensuring that you are not taking a supplement or medication that contains any of the banned substances. The United States Anti-Doping Agency keeps an updated list on what is currently banned in the United States. If you are prescribed a medication that contains a banned substance, you can file for a therapeutic use exemption.

Supplements

The Dietary Supplement Health and Education Act of 1994 (DSHEA) defined a supplement as a nonfood, a nonfood additive, and a nondrug, so that supplements would not fall under the same stringent restrictions as foods. While the FDA has the ability to remove products that have been shown to cause health issues, there are no strict guidelines for production, quality, and content. This act also allows supplement companies to make claims without scientific proof and to be intentionally vague. As long as supplement companies do not claim to cure or mitigate a disease, they can make any unsubstantiated claim they desire. The DSHEA allows supplements to remain outside of good manufacturing practices (GMP), which require that all drugs be within a very strict limit (typically within 1 to 2 percent) of what is stated on the label. Because supplements are not regulated by the FDA for content, many products do not contain the exact amount of the stated ingredient in the product. Scientific studies have examined supplements and found that some have exactly what is stated on the package while others have little to none of the advertised product.

Due to the way supplements are marketed, it can be difficult to know what works and what does not. This makes it difficult to determine if a specific product will work as advertised, and it is important to look to other sources for information. Sometimes the testimonies of professional athletes are sought out as sources. But beware, often professional athletes are paid by the supplement companies to advertise products. The athlete may or may not actually use the product in training, however, and may even just believe that the supplement works when it truly has no effect on performance.

Magazines are also not a valid source for information on the effects of ergogenic aids. The magazine may be reluctant to print an article that a supplement does not work when that company is paying for advertising in its pages. It is not uncommon to see a supplement advertisement appearing as an article and then in tiny print somewhere on the page stating that it is a paid advertisement.

Peer-reviewed scientific journal articles are the best sources of information because the reviewed studies are conducted under strictly controlled settings and in an unbiased manner. This can be difficult at times due to not having free access to all journals, and they are often written in such a way that you need a strong understanding of chemistry to know what is stated in the article. Textbooks are often a good source as they have condensed the information from various scientific articles into an understandable review of the ergogenic aid.

If you decide to try a specific ergogenic aid, ensure that you know the possible side effects, and pay attention to how your body reacts to the supplement. Most supplements are expensive; you do not want to waste money on something that will not work for you. Calculate a cost benefit ratio for yourself.

There are a few ergogenic aids that can be beneficial for obstacle course racing. Some were mentioned at the beginning of the chapter (water, carbohydrates, proteins, and sports drinks). If you do not think water is an ergogenic aid, try running on a hot day without it and see what happens to your performance (joking, don't do that). Protein is also a vital ergogenic aid as it greatly assists in the anabolic process in the body, aiding in recovery. Carbohydrate ingestion during competition has been shown to improve performance during sustained endurance events and is vital for refueling during recovery. Electrolyte replacement is also vital during long events and for recovery. One common ergogenic aid that we have not discussed is caffeine.

Caffeine

Believe it or not, caffeine is also an ergogenic aid and is the most widely used supplement in the world. It is a naturally occurring stimulant found in plants (coffee beans, tea leaves, cocoa nuts, etc.). Caffeine is also found naturally in many products we use daily, such as coffee, tea, and soda, but it is often added to other products as a stimulant. Research strongly supports the use of caffeine for improving human performance during endurance sports.

Caffeine can improve performance in three basic ways. The first is that it can easily cross the blood/brain barrier, acting as an ergogenic aid by decreasing feelings of pain and fatigue during exercise, resulting in the ability to race or train at a higher intensity level. The second is that caffeine both stimulates and increases the mobilization of free fatty acids into the blood, resulting in an increased availability for energy production and, thus, conserving glycogen stores. And finally, caffeine increases the muscles' ability to contract by also increasing activity at the neuromuscular junction and increasing motor unit recruitment.

While caffeine is widely used by a large portion of the population, there are potential side effects. The most common include muscle tremors, gastrointestinal distress, headache, nervousness, elevated heart rate, arrhythmia, and high blood pressure. Side effects are more likely to develop at high levels of ingestion and in individuals who do not normally consume caffeine. While it is commonly stated that caffeine acts as a diuretic, research has shown that this is not true during exercise, primarily due to the release of anti-diuretic hormone and aldosterone that occurs during exercise in order to retain water. The risk of dehydration and thermoregulatory complications is more likely to occur with caffeine ingestion in a hot environment.

It is important to know how your body reacts to caffeine prior to using it as an ergogenic aid, and it should never be used in high dosages. In fact, caffeine does not have to be taken in large doses to increase endurance performance. Caffeine ingestion equivalent to 2.5 cups of coffee has been found to be sufficient to improve performance. Caffeine peaks in the system around one hour after ingestion and therefore should be taken an hour prior to competition. Also be aware that some organizations consider caffeine a banned substance. The NCAA bans caffeine usage equivalent to about six to nine 8-ounce cups of coffee. The number of cups will vary depending on the athlete's body mass and timing of ingestion. Do not take caffeine pills as the quantity of caffeine within a pill is suspect. Anecdotally, I have worked with athletes who were habitual coffee drinkers that experienced negative health consequences when using caffeine pills as an ergogenic aid.

Habitual use of caffeine actually diminishes its ergogenic effect. For those who ingest caffeine (coffee, soda, etc.) on a regular basis, it is recommended to cease caffeine consumption seven days prior to competition in order to optimize the effects of caffeine for sports performance.

Anabolic Steroids

Two illegal ergogenic aids that are commonly used in OCR are anabolic steroids and blood doping. This and the next section will discuss both of these ergogenic aids to give you a better understanding of how they work and why you should avoid their use. It is also important to educate yourself on these topics as they are often discussed in relation to training and competing in elite-level sports.

Anabolic steroids (synthetic testosterone) are unfortunately prevalent in all sports. Steroids promote the anabolic process in the body and improve performance by increasing the speed of recovery, repairing damaged tissue, creating greater hypertrophy, and reducing the catabolic effects of exercise. The ability to recover faster between training bouts allows an athlete to train harder more often, which in turn leads to improved performance. Steroids are typically administered through injection, oral doses, patches, or cream.

There are reversible and irreversible side effects that occur with steroid use. Reversible side effects include acne, depression, increased rage, infections at injection sites, and high cholesterol. These side effects dissipate once steroid use has stopped.

The irreversible side effects of steroids occur due to prolonged and heavy use and are typically more serious. They include cancer, liver disease, cardiovascular disease, and baldness. Side effects that are specific to males are testicular atrophy, impotence, developing mammary glands (breasts), and a permanent decrease in natural testosterone production. Women run the risk of developing facial hair and a deeper voice. Steroid use in pregnant women can also lead to birth defects. Due to the lack of strong scientific research studies in humans, it is not possible to truly know all the negative impacts steroid use has on health.

Blood Doping

The term "blood doping" covers any method used to increase red blood cell count. Red blood cells are responsible for transport of oxygen, which is a key component for endurance sports. If red blood cells increase, then your ability to transport oxygen to the working muscles also increases, and therefore endurance performance increases. There are three primary methods used for blood doping: autologous, homologous, and erythropoietin. Autologous blood doping involves removing blood from the athlete and spinning the blood in order to separate plasma from hemoglobin. The plasma is then injected back into the athlete and the red blood cells are stored for later use. It takes approximately four to six weeks for hemoglobin levels to return to normal. The hemoglobin is then reinfused prior to competition in order to increase red blood cell count. The downside to this method is that the athlete will be weak for a period of time, which affects training.

To prevent the period of weakness following blood removal during autologous blood doping, some athletes choose to use homologous blood doping instead. Homologous blood doping involves infusing red blood cells from a matched donor just prior to racing. This method carries a high risk of disease transmission and infection, and it is possible that the athlete's body may reject the donor blood. Antigens found in blood differ significantly between individuals, making this method of blood doping easy to detect.

Erythropoietin is a naturally occurring hormone that is produced in the kidneys and is responsible for stimulating red blood cell production in the bone marrow. Epoetin (synthetic erythropoietin) is injected in order to increase red blood cell production. A negative side effect of epoetin is that it can drastically increase red blood cell production, resulting in a large increase in hematocrit, which can negatively impact health. The use of epoetin also requires iron supplementation in order to provide the excess iron needed to create hemoglobin.

Blood doping is banned not only because it gives the athlete an unfair advantage but also due to the serious health complications that can occur when implementing this process. All three of these methods significantly increase hematocrit levels. If hematocrit gets too high, it will result in an increase in blood viscosity, which in turn could lead to a stroke or heart attack. Obstacle course racing requires endurance performance over a prolonged period, and on a hot day dehydration can easily occur. When an athlete becomes dehydrated, plasma volumes are significantly decreased, which increases blood viscosity. Blood doping combined with dehydration is a deadly formula.

6

COMPETITION

As mentioned previously, the first step in developing your training plan is to determine your race schedule. In this section I am going to discuss where and how to find races. Obstacle course races are expensive to organize and require a lot of work; therefore, you will most likely find very few local races throughout the season and should be willing to travel in order to race. To find any local obstacle course races, contact the local running clubs and running shops. They typically have information on when and where local races occur.

One good way to find upcoming races is to research the major obstacle race promoters. At the time of writing this book, the major race promoters are Spartan, Tough Mudder, and Rugged Maniac. Promoters have come and gone in this field, so the list may change as you are reading this book. Visit their websites to see when and where all their races are held each year. These race promoters put on well-organized, well-supported, and safe races.

Active.com is another internet source for obstacle course race information, from the big names to your local events. On Active.com, choose obstacle course racing from a drop-down menu as they are a registration site for many different sports. You can then search by your location in order to find races that are close to you.

Obstacle course races are held at varying distances and through varying terrain, and it is important to know both in order to make a decision on whether or not to add the race to your schedule. If you are new to obstacle course racing, keep the distances lower and carefully pick your terrain. For example, there is a difference between a 5k obstacle course race on relatively flat land and one conducted on the slope of a mountain. Some race promoters will have races during the same weekend that can range from a 5k to a half marathon. Make sure to choose the appropriate distance for your predicted fitness level.

The size of the race may be something you want to consider as well. Some racers prefer smaller events with smaller crowds and fewer racers, whereas other competitors prefer large crowds and a large race field. Both have their advantages and disadvantages. The smaller races have fewer people and therefore are typically less crowded on the course. A smaller group of people racing may also be less intimidating for those just starting out. The downside to smaller races is that they may not be as well supported on the course. Large races have a big wow factor that brings with it a lot of excitement and energy. When you have 1,000-plus athletes competing in an event, it creates a festive atmosphere that takes on a life of its own, providing a great experience for everyone involved.

REGISTRATION

You can save money by registering early for races. At times these savings can be very substantial. Make sure to note the fee-increase dates so that you do not miss the lower early-entry costs. Early registration also guarantees you a spot in popular races. Some races fill up quickly, and if you wait too long you will not be able to obtain a spot to race or you may be limited on choosing a start time that works for you. A downside to early registration is that very few races will refund registration fees if you find it necessary to back out for any reason. However, some do allow racers to transfer their registration to another race, at a cost.

LOGISTICS

When choosing a race, also consider the logistical requirements (scheduling, travel, and lodging). Ensure that the date will fit within your current family schedule, work schedule, and training schedule. Always double-check your calendar prior to registration so that you do not double book. While some race promoters will allow you to transfer your race fees to another race (at a cost), most registration fees are nonrefundable.

Next, determine the distance you will have to travel in order to compete. Local travel is usually very easy as you can arrive at the race in the morning, compete, and then return home. The farther the race is from your home, the more planning you must do. You may need to travel a day or two prior to the race and will need to decide if you are driving or flying, as well as make hotel arrangements. Local races are typically less expensive (no lodging and minimal travel), require less planning, and are typically less stressful overall. If you are flying to the race, consider ground transportation at your destination as well.

Prior to race weekend, review the race schedule and plan your weekend based on that. Determine when and where packet pickup will occur, and schedule accordingly. Most races have packet pickup the morning of the race near the start time. However, some races require packet pickup the day prior to the race, which may or may not be at the race site. Most races will have packet pickup both on the day prior and on race day. Picking up your packet the day before the race allows you to make sure everything is good with your registration. Take the time to read through the race material for any specialized information concerning the race and pay close attention to your race day and start time. I have seen racers miss their start time or show up on the wrong day to race.

Race Budget

Develop a budget for your registration fees, travel, and lodging. Race fees are not inexpensive and can add up quickly as the race season progresses. Entry fees for obstacle course races range from $35 to over $200. Make a list of your chosen races with the cost for each. Then add travel, lodging, and food costs into your budget for each race. This will give you an outline for your race season budget. Once you know how much you will spend in the upcoming race season, you can then develop a plan to meet the budget requirements for racing.

Equipment Check

The night before you leave for a race, conduct an equipment check to ensure you have everything you need. You do not want to show up to a race minus your running shoes or any other vital equipment. Create a checklist with everything you will need before, during, and after the race. The next step is to lay out all your gear and visually mark everything off the list. The biggest mistake people can make here is to not see their equipment and yet check it off the list, thinking an item is still in their race bag and forgetting it was taken out last week for cleaning. If you arrive at a race without something you need, however, large race venues will typically have sales tents with about every piece of equipment needed for a race, but it will not be cheap, and you will then be racing in a piece of equipment that has not been worn in prior races. Below is a basic checklist of the equipment you will need for most obstacle course races. Adjust the checklist to fit your specific needs.

- race shoes
- post-race shoes (Crocs are great for this)
- race clothes (top, bottom, socks, head gear, whatever you are racing in)
- post-race clothing
- two towels (one for mud and the other to dry off after you are clean)
- nutrition (for before, during, and after the race)
- registration information
- cash (for parking fee or anything you may need to buy from the race venue)
- photo ID (some races require photo ID at packet pickup)
- bag for muddy clothes (trash bag, dry bag, etc.)
- first-aid kit
- hydration pack (essential for long races)
- toiletries (soap, deodorant, anything needed for cleanup after the race)
- clothing for any inclement weather

If you are going to be gone for more than one day, you may want to consider packing two bags. The first bag is your race bag for all your racing gear and tools. The second bag will contain clothing, travel supplies, and anything else you may need. If you are flying, however, you may not want two separate bags due to cost. If you can avoid it, do not check your race bag as the airlines are known for lost baggage.

Race Day

On race day get up early enough to eat, go to the bathroom, and arrive at the race venue with plenty of time to line up for the start of the race. Get to the race venue early enough to find parking, ensure you are geared up and ready, conduct your warm-up, and line up at the start line on time. Getting there early allows you to prepare for the race without the extra anxiety of rushing and worrying about missing your start time.

If you were unable to pick up your race packet prior to race day, this should be your first stop of the morning to ensure that there are no unforeseen complications and because the lines can be long. If the event uses timing chips, place those on your shoe, wrist, or ankle. I prefer the wrist so that there is less worry about it coming loose while traversing obstacles. Double-check the start time and start location of your specific race as there are multiple start waves.

Now that you have everything set up to race, you will most likely need to find the bathroom prior to beginning your warm-up. Unfortunately, when you are nervous about the race it is inevitable that you will require another bathroom stop. As there are always many more racers and spectators than bathrooms, it is a good idea to get that out of the way early as well. Don't make the mistake of having to decide whether to remain in the bathroom line or start the race.

Next is your warm-up. Make sure that you time your warm-up so that you are ready to go at your appropriate start time. Do not warm up for too long or too early if you have a later start time. The actual race course will most likely be closed prior to the start, and you may have to warm up on the road or on an alternate trail. I prefer doing short loops for my warm-up and not going too far from the start so that I do not miss anything.

TYPES OF OBSTACLES

Overhead Obstacles

Overhead obstacles are a staple of OCR; therefore, it is important to work on this unique skill in order to perform well during a race. Overhead obstacles usually consist of an overhead rig with various hanging mechanisms you must cross hand over hand while suspended in the air. The most common mechanisms are rings, dial rods, bars, ropes, and swinging bars. An overhead obstacle can be as simple as monkey bars or as complex as a mixture of mechanisms on the same rig. Traversing overhead obstacles is not a natural locomotive pattern and therefore must be practiced. This section will cover a few basic concepts that will help you better compete in this area.

The foundation of successful overhead obstacle skill is the muscular endurance of your core, upper body, and grip (forearms and hands). If you do not have the muscular endurance base to accomplish the task, then your skill will not matter. The best way to provide this base is through a solid strength-and-conditioning program that includes pull-ups, lat pull-downs, and overhead obstacles. Climbing is another way to improve upper body muscular endurance. If you have a climbing gym in your area, give it a try.

Swinging

When working swinging obstacles (see fig. 6.1) such as ropes, rings, or dials, there are a few key concepts to remember. I will only discuss rings in this section, but all comments will hold true for most swinging obstacles. The first key concept involves having two hands holding your body weight at all times. When swinging from ring to ring, do not let go of one ring and swing that same hand

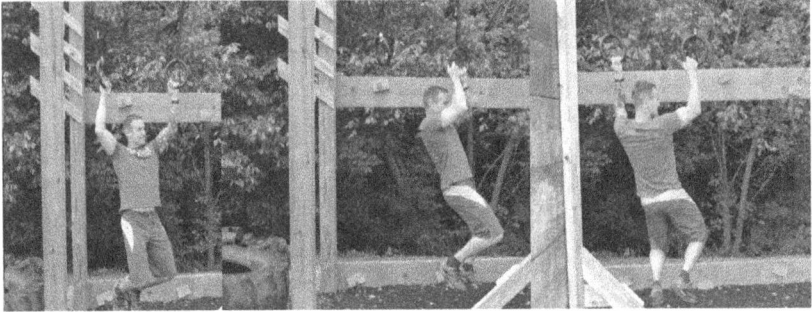

Figure 6.1. Swinging obstacles. *Grayson Peveler.*

forward past the ring in your other hand to the next ring. Instead, when you let go of the ring, grab the same ring you are holding with your other hand. As you swing forward, grab the next ring. Make sure that you have a firm grip prior to releasing the other hand. With this method, there will be a brief second where you are only holding on with one hand. Not only is this method less fatiguing, but the main benefit is that it greatly reduces the chances of your hand slipping in wet, muddy conditions.

Next is to swing correctly. To get your momentum going, bend your back arm, which will swing you backward, and then straighten your back arm to swing forward. As you come forward, bend your front arm to help pull you forward. As you straighten your front arm, you will start to go backward. Use this method to gain the momentum you need to swing forward. Before releasing your back hand, make sure you are swinging in a straight line toward the next ring. If you are at an angle, you may not be able to reach the ring, leaving you stuck on one ring at an angle that will make it impossible to move forward or back.

Another important concept is to keep your movements smooth and your momentum going throughout the obstacles. Jerky movements make it more difficult to progress and more likely that you will slip on an obstacle. In addition, keeping a rhythm and maintaining your momentum will require less energy to complete the task. Hesitation between obstacles will require more time and energy to regain your momentum, resulting in greater upper body fatigue and decrease in grip strength.

Rotating

On the overhead rig there may be objects that rotate or move as you traverse the obstacle. When working these holds, maintain a secure handhold with both hands and shift your weight as the object rotates. The Spartan twister is an example of a rotating-handhold obstacle. In this obstacle there is a long metal pole with offset handles. As you grab a handle, the pole rotates downward with your weight. To successfully complete this obstacle, make sure that you have two hands on the obstacle as often as possible. There are two ways to complete this obstacle. The first is to face the bar sideways so that every time you grab a handhold, the bar rotates toward you and you progress sideways across the twister. The other way is to travel backward in line with the pole, reaching behind your head for each handhold. Conducting this backward may seem a little awkward until you try it. Practice both methods to see which works best for you.

Regardless of the method you choose, one key concept will remain the same: when you grab a new hold do not let go with your other hand until the new handhold is at the bottom, you have a firm grip, and you start to swing forward. When you reach forward and grab a new handhold, it is offset from your current handhold, which is now vertical. So when you grab the new handhold and transfer your weight to it, that handhold will begin to drop to vertical while your previous handhold leaves the vertical position. Do not release your previous handhold until the new handhold is vertical and your weight is moving forward. If you release your first hold early, the new handhold will drop quickly and may cause you to slip. While you want to be cautious, do not move slowly as this will result in fatigue prior to reaching the other side. Instead, work on moving in a rhythm that will get you across without the risk of slipping or fatigue.

Monkey Bars

The monkey bars are another variation of the overhead obstacles you will encounter (see fig. 6.2). There are various methods to use here. Most people have used the simple swing when traversing monkey bars as a kid. Swing forward and grab the bar with one hand, release the back hand, and swing forward using your momentum to the next bar. This is a quick, easy method to traverse the monkey bars. However, there is a high risk of slipping if the bars are wet or muddy.

Another method is to move each hand to a single bar as you move forward. This method minimizes the time that you do not have two hands on the bar and makes it less likely that you will slip. For this method you will keep your arms slightly bent and drive the leg on the side of the hand you want to advance forward as you release to grab the bar. Once you are secure you will drive your other leg forward as well as your hand to grab the same bar. You will progress

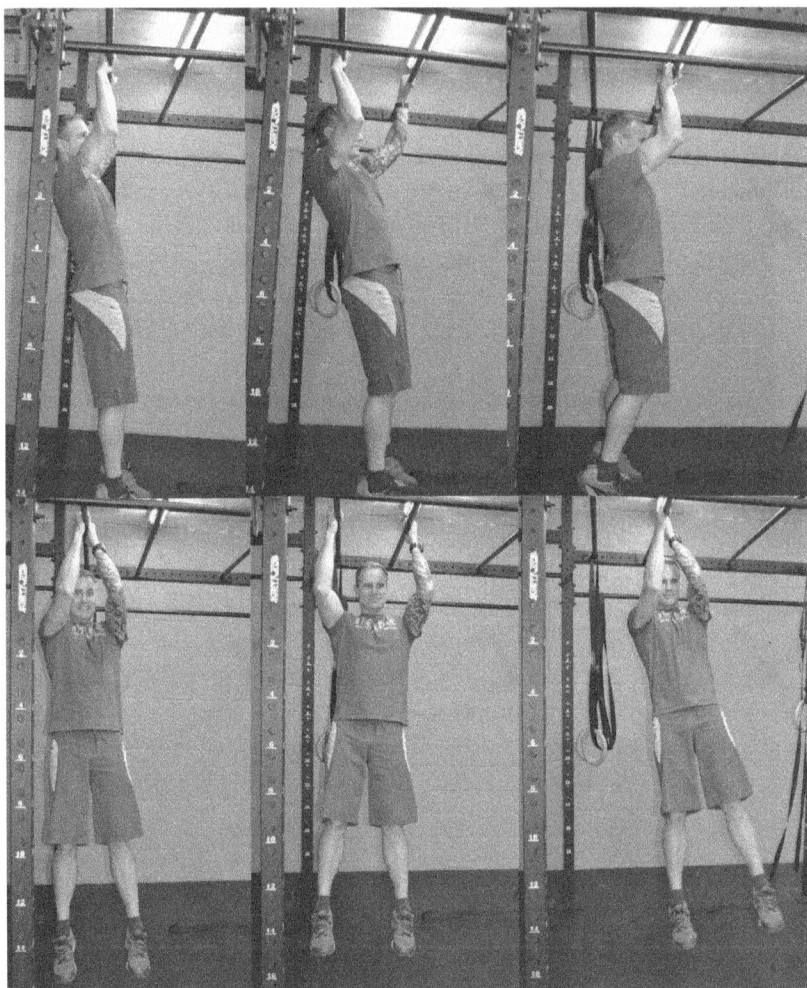

Figure 6.2. Monkey bars. *Grayson Peveler.*

across the bar in this manner. While it is more secure than the swing method, it does take a little longer.

The last method is the sideways method. This method provides the best grip in wet or muddy conditions. Stand under the bar with your right shoulder facing the direction you want to travel. Jump up and grab the bar with your left hand just in front of your right hand. The back of your right hand and the palm of your left hand should both face the direction of travel. Slightly bend your arms and then swing from your hips and reach out to grab the next bar with your right hand, keeping the back of the hand facing the direction of travel. Next bring your left hand to the bar with your palm facing the direction you are traveling. Complete this process across the monkey bars.

Military Rope Bridge

The military rope bridge is a rope that is pulled tight between two objects. You will be required to travel across the rope without touching the ground. There are multiple ways to cross the rope as you can cross it on top or underneath. I am not going to discuss the on-top method as there is a lot of friction created while traversing, and chances are you will not be dressed to prevent rope burn. This method also requires greater balance and is slower.

The method for crossing underneath the rope bridge begins with your back facing the direction you want to travel. Grab the rope with both hands and lift your legs up and cross them over the rope. If you have socks on, you can just keep your legs locked and pull yourself hand over hand across the rope. If you do not have socks on, then you will get rope burns using this method and will need to make a slight adjustment.

To avoid rope burns, alternate legs on the rope so that they do not slide along the rope as you travel. Start with both hands and both legs locked onto the rope. Next reach forward with your right hand and bring your left knee forward at the same time. At this point your left hand and right leg are locked onto the rope, providing a strong base. As you grab the rope with your right hand, lock your left leg across the rope while moving your right leg out of the way and forward as you now reach forward with your left hand. Repeat this process across the rope. It is important to lock in with one leg before moving the other leg and to lock in with one hand prior to releasing the other. With practice you will develop a rhythm that will get you across the rope quickly and with less effort.

Climbing Obstacles

There will be many climbing obstacles during an obstacle course race. As with the overhead obstacles, muscular endurance of the core, upper body, and grip will be needed here. However, for climbing you will also use the lower body. While muscular endurance is necessary, applying the correct technique will result in faster and more efficient climbs. There are particular skills required to quickly and effectively climb the various obstacles. This section will touch on a few of those skills.

Rope

The rope climb (see fig. 6.3) is much more challenging than it seems. The trick to easily climbing the rope is to use the correct technique. Beginners make the mistake of climbing the rope using all upper body strength. While this can be accomplished, it requires a much greater use of energy than is necessary and takes longer. The correct way to climb a rope is to utilize your legs.

The two most common methods for climbing a rope are called the J hook and the S hook (or S wrap). Practice both and see which you are most comfortable with. In this section, I will discuss both methods. Before you begin climbing to the top of a rope, however, practice your chosen climbing method until you are able to hang on the rope without placing weight on your arms and your legs and feet are solidly engaged. Once you can accomplish this task, then start using the method to climb.

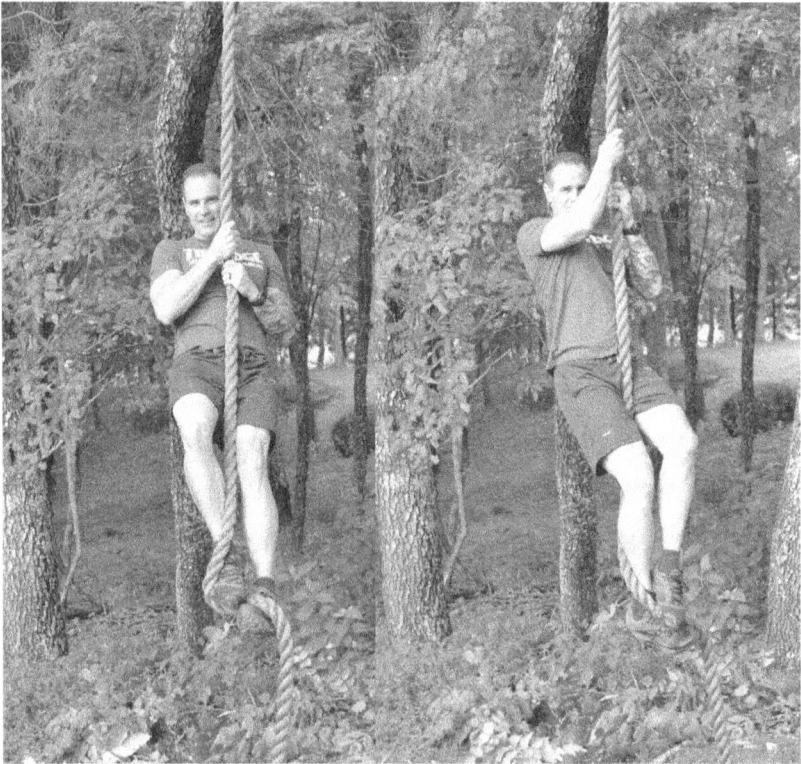

Figure 6.3. Rope climb, J- and S-hook methods. *Grayson Peveler.*

To use the J hook method, jump or reach up as high as you can and grab the rope. Jumping allows you to start higher on the rope, but may not be recommended if the rope is caked in mud. Lift your legs and feet into the air so that your knees are near your chest. As you bring your legs up, make sure the rope is on the outside of your right foot. Grab the rope with your left foot just below your right foot and bring the rope across the bottom of your right foot. As you do so, make sure that the rope also stays to the outside of that foot. Bring the rope up the inside of your right foot and slightly cross your left foot over your right, locking the rope in place. Once you are locked in, push up with your legs and walk your hands up the rope as your legs extend. Once our legs are fully extended and your hands are as high as possible, grip the rope, lift your knees toward your chest again, and repeat the process.

Once you reach the top, you will have to descend. Be careful on the descent as descending too quickly or with too tight a grip can cause friction burns on your hands. To descend, work your way down hand over hand while supporting your weight with your legs. Loosen the grip on the rope with your feet and control the speed of your descent by allowing the rope to glide through your feet.

To use the S hook method, begin by jumping or reaching up as high as you can and grab the rope. Lift your legs and feet into the air so that your knees are near your chest. With the rope between your legs, wrap the rope around your right calf and across the top of your foot. Place your left foot on top of the rope and on top of your right foot, locking the rope in place. Once you lock the rope in place with your feet, extend your legs and walk your hands up the rope doing all the work with your legs. Keeping the rope in place, loosen your grip with your feet and bring your legs up to your chest and repeat the process. To descend, loosen the grip with your feet, allowing the rope to slide in between, and walk your hands down the rope.

The process of climbing a rope becomes increasingly difficult when you factor in mud. Before attempting the climb, make sure that your hands are dry and clear of mud as wet, muddy hands make it more difficult to maintain a secure grip. Knock as much mud off your shoes as you can before you start as well. If you are racing later in the day, the lower part of the rope will most likely be caked in mud by the time you reach it. If the rope is clear of mud higher up, then jump and grab the dry area and bring your legs up and lock them in place. If the rope is muddy higher than you can jump, then you should avoid jumping as you will most likely slip when you grab the rope. Instead, clear mud from the rope at the point you plan on grabbing and begin your climb from that point.

Vertical Cargo Net

Another common climbing obstacle is the vertical cargo net, which can be tricky. The difficulty is due to the way the cargo net is set up. It is hung high between two poles or trees. The upper wire is pulled tight horizontally and the cargo net hangs down vertically to the ground with plenty of slack lying on the ground. The lack of vertical tension is what makes the climb challenging; if vertical tension were placed on the cargo net, making it tight, then it would not be much different than climbing a metal ladder. The lack of vertical tension requires greater balance, strength, and skill to climb. There are a few tricks that will make your climb go much more smoothly.

The first is to pick your climbing path. Choose one vertical rope line up and use that line for climbing. When climbing, place your hands on the vertical rope line going up and not on the horizontal rope lines. This keeps your balance centered and the tension on that one rope line. When grabbing the rope line, grasp just above where the vertical and horizontal lines meet so that you are not using a large amount of grip strength as you climb. Place your feet on the horizontal rope line right next to the vertical rope line you are gripping with your hands. This placement of your hands and feet will provide a more downward-directed force on the one line and reduce horizontal displacement as you climb.

For many OCR competitors, crossing the top of the vertical cargo net is the scariest part because they feel like they have little to no control. There are numerous ways to cross. You will see professional racers reach both arms over the top and then reach down and grab a horizontal rope. From this point, they just flip over the top. It is fast and effective, but not ideal for beginning racers. The easiest way to alleviate this fear is to make sure that you have control when you reach the top of the net. At the top, focus on the tension line that runs between the two poles as it will not move much. Then slip your right arm over the top, grabbing the net on the other side with the top rope firmly under your armpit. Grab the top with your left hand. Once both hands are secured, bring your right leg up and over. Begin to move your body toward the top and hook your right leg in on the back side of the cargo net. Once your right leg is secured, begin to shift your weight to that leg, controlling the motion with your hands as well. Once you are supporting your weight with your hands and body on the top rope and with your right leg on the back side of the cargo net, begin to move your body and the other leg over the top and to the back side of the cargo net. Then climb down the same way you climbed up.

Wall Climb

Wall climbs are another common obstacle you will encounter when racing. Wall height varies, however, so you will need to plan your attack based on the height of the wall in each race. For walls on which you can easily reach the top by just grabbing it or by a small jump, there are three easy ways to go over the wall. The first is for beginners, those who are tired, or those with less upper body strength. Begin by facing the wall; grab and hold the top. Turn your body toward your left arm and bring your left foot to the top of the wall, hooking the top with your heel. Using your leg and arms bring your body up toward the top of the wall. Allow your left leg to go over the top and sit straddled on the wall. Shift your weight to your hands with your body facing the way you just came and swing your right leg over. Next just lower yourself to the ground. (See fig. 6.4.)

Another method involves placing your hands on the top of the wall, jumping up, and extending your arms until they are straight. If your timing is good, you will conduct this movement fluidly as you run up to the wall, which also helps with the upward motion of this movement. From this position, bring your left leg up and place your foot with the sole down on the top of the wall. You can then use your leg and arms to bring your body weight upward. At this point, swing your right foot over the wall and jump down to the other side.

The last common method for climbing a wall is to lean over the wall with your upper body. This one takes a little more skill in order to prevent landing on your head. The initial approach to the wall is similar to the last method. Place your hands on the top of the wall, jump, and push up with your arms. When

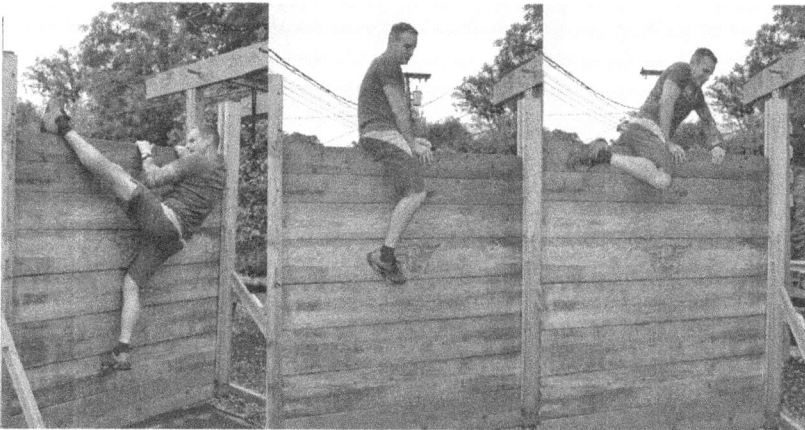

Figure 6.4. **Wall climb.** *Grayson Peveler.*

enough of your body is above the top of the wall so that you can lean over at the waist, do so, placing your weight on the top of the wall at your waist. Allow your right hand to move to the back side of the wall and brace against the wall. Your left hand will drop to the front of the wall. You will brace with both hands, preventing you from completely toppling over the wall and onto the ground. At the same time you are bracing with your hands, both legs are coming up and over the wall, using your waist as a pivot point. Bring your feet below you and land.

When you are tackling taller walls, such as an 8- or 10-foot wall, your approach will change. Momentum and timing are key aspects when it comes to scaling larger walls. If you are taller or can jump well, you may be able to just stand or jump up and grab the wall, similar to what I discussed previously. However, if you cannot jump well or are vertically challenged, then you must adjust your approach. Before attempting this climb, make sure that you have as much mud off the bottom of your shoes as possible.

The first thing to do is build momentum. The greater your momentum, the higher you will be able to go. Your momentum will add to the normal reaction force that will occur between your foot and the wall, which in turn greatly increases the necessary friction there. Next, time your jump so that you leave the ground about 2 to 3 feet away from the wall. If you jump too close to the wall, you will not have the proper angle to redirect your momentum upward toward the top of the wall. Jump so that your right foot makes contact with the wall while you are in the air. Your left hand will also make contact with the wall in order to prevent your upper body from flying too far forward and to assist with directing momentum upward. When your right foot makes contact with the wall, push hard downward in order to accelerate upward. Reach high with your right arm to grab the top as you push down with your right foot. Grab the wall with your right hand and then your left. Once both hands have secure holds on the top of the wall, you can use one of the previous methods discussed to get over the top.

Carrying Obstacles

Another common category of obstacles that you will find at a race is the carry. The carry is just as it sounds: you will be required to carry a weighted object over a fixed distance. In most races there will be different weights for males and females. Some of the common objects you will find yourself carrying are the buckets, sandbags, logs, atlas stones, and concrete blocks. It requires muscular strength and muscular endurance to accomplish this task, so be sure to include weighted carry within your normal training program. Like most sports, movement techniques are a vital component of success. Knowing the correct techniques for each carry will go a long way toward assisting you in completing these obstacles in a timely and efficient manner. I will discuss a few basic techniques for the bucket and sandbag carries. These same methods can be used for other basic carries.

Bucket

The bucket carry is a common obstacle that you will encounter in OCR. The buckets used are typical 5-gallon paint buckets. If you want to practice for the bucket carry, you can purchase a 5-gallon bucket from your local hardware store. In some races you are required to fill the bucket and then carry it a fixed distance. If you have to fill your own bucket, make sure that you fill it a little past the full line as the contents will settle or spill as you move through that section of the course. You do not want to carry the heavy bucket all the way to the end and then find out you failed the obstacle because your bucket was not full.

The first key point here is to lift with your legs and not your back. Never bend over to pick up the bucket. To begin, squat down with the bucket between your legs and slightly forward. Do not bend forward over the bucket as this will put undue strain on your back. Grab the bucket and stand using your legs and hips.

There are a few grips you can use to carry the bucket. But, first, it is important to mention that you should not grab the bucket at the bottom with both hands as your hands will want to slide to the outside of the bucket, and this will exhaust your grip quickly. Instead, choose one of the following grips. The first is the bear hug. Wrap your arms around the bucket and grab your wrist. Or you could hold the bottom of the bucket with one hand, and with the other hand grab the wrist and top of the hand that is grasping the bottom of the bucket. Practice with both of these grips and see which you prefer. On long bucket carries, you may need to switch your grip from time to time. If the rules allow it, you can carry the bucket on your shoulder.

If you need to rest, go to one knee and set the bucket on the quadriceps of the leg that is parallel to the ground. This allows you to rest your grip without setting the bucket all the way on the ground, which will save you some energy.

Sandbag

The sandbag carry requires you to carry a weighted sandbag over a fixed distance. The sandbags vary in size, shape, and weight from race to race. With the sandbag carry, it's best to carry the bag on your shoulders as opposed to with your arms.

If the bag is long enough, drape it across your upper back and hold both ends with your hands, allowing your back to take the weight. While your hands and arms will have to work to balance the bag and keep it in place, most of the weight should be supported across your back and shoulders. Small sandbags make this method difficult, however. In that case, place the sandbag across one shoulder and balance it with that arm, but be sure to switch shoulders prior to becoming fatigued, which will also help to maintain your kinetic balance.

Atlas Stone

Atlas stone carries (see fig. 6.5) are also used in obstacle course racing. Due to the weight and shape of the atlas stone, the carries are much shorter than either the bucket or sandbag carry in competition. The hardest part about the atlas stone carry is the pickup. There are two common methods. The first is used by strongmen competitors when lifting and training. However, the stones used in obstacle course racing are significantly lighter than those used in strongman competitions, so there is also an alternative method. Try both and see which works best for your particular strength level and anthropometrics.

To pick up the atlas stone, place your feet on each side of the stone with the center line of the stone just in front of your shins and in line with the ball of your feet. You want the stone as close to you as possible while still being able to lift it. The farther away the stone's center of mass is from your center of mass, the harder it will be to lift and the greater the risk of injury. Your feet should be close to the stone so that as you pick it up, you can set the stone on your quadriceps (discussed below). If your feet are set too wide, the stone will slip between your legs instead.

Once your feet are set, squat down and place your hands under the stone keeping your arms almost straight with only a slight bend. If your arms are bent too much, you will be placing unnecessary strain on the muscles of the arms, which can result in early fatigue. Your fingers should be spread in order to help increase your grip on the stone. Do not drop your bottom hand down into a deep squat as this will put you out of proper position for a good lift.

Lift the stone, and as soon as you are past your knees, squat low and roll the stone onto your quadriceps, giving the stone support and allowing you to adjust your grip. A common mistake is to attempt to keep the stone from touching your legs as you come up, because it is uncomfortable, but this places the stone too far from the body. Once the stone is on your quadriceps, move your

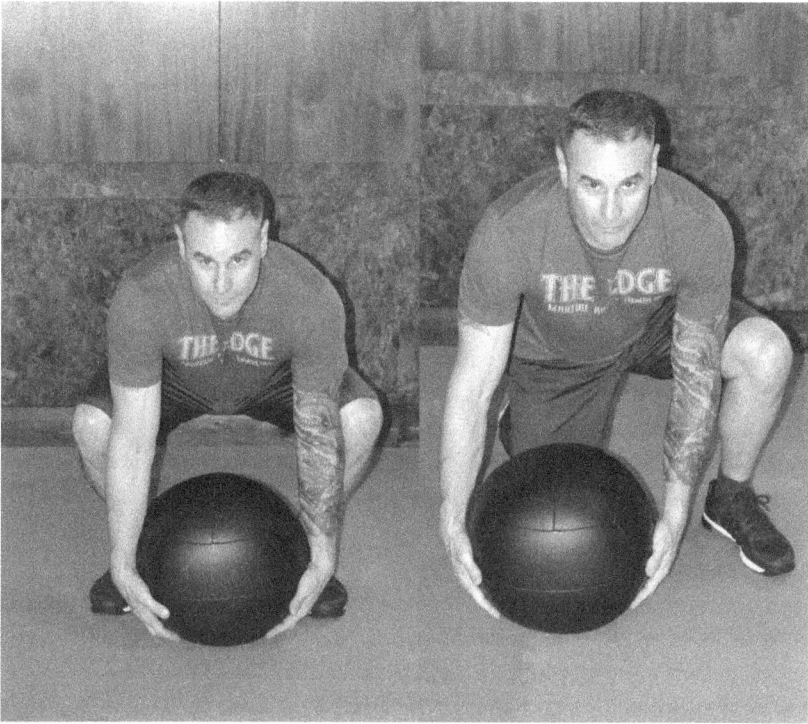

Figure 6.5.   Atlas stone, two-leg and one-leg pickup. *Will and Renee Peveler.*

hands forward to a comfortable position and then stand up, using your legs. As the atlas stone moves up your body, make sure to keep it close and do not push it out.

The second method works particularly well in OCR competitions due to the lighter weight of the stones used, but it does require more strength during the pickup. Begin by kneeling down with one knee on the ground. The knee that is on the ground should be centered behind the atlas stone. Grab the stone with both hands, with your fingers spread apart to increase friction. Once you are set, roll or scoop the stone onto the quadriceps of the knee that is on the ground. Once the stone is securely in place, stand using your legs and move the stone into the carry position.

Low Obstacles

Obstacle course races will have at least one obstacle that will require you to low-crawl under or through an object for a short distance. This is why it is important to include the army crawl, alligator crawl, and bear crawl in your training. These exercises will ensure that you have good muscular strength and core stability, and a good range of motion. Common low obstacles used in these races are barbed wire, rope, netting, wood, and tunnels.

The barbed-wire crawl is the most common. This obstacle will require the low crawl or a variation of it. The army low crawl is ideal for this situation as it keeps the body close to the ground and away from the obstacle. Body awareness is important when traveling under low obstacles. Always know where your body is in relation to the obstacle to prevent being snagged by the barbs.

The fundamental techniques of the army crawl were discussed in chapter 3. Reread that section if you need a review. As you are performing the army crawl, do not roll up on your side when you bring your knee forward as it may push your hip into the obstacle overhead. If your hips roll up during this movement, work on your flexibility until you can bring your knee forward without rolling your hips up. Your hips should stay relatively flat to the ground as your knee comes forward. Keep your head and shoulders low as well. Many beginners will raise their heads and upper bodies, which then get snagged on the barbs.

It is vital to train for low obstacles. The barbed-wire crawl can be anywhere from 100 to over 200 feet in length, which is a long way to crawl. If you do not have the muscular endurance to crawl that far, your muscles will fatigue and cramp during the crawl and you may lack the necessary flexibility in that position. Make sure that you can comfortably cover the distance at home before racing.

Also, do not attempt to roll under the barbed-wire obstacle. Though some racers can successfully perform the roll, it is not ideal for most racers. The main reason to avoid this is that you will become dizzy and start feeling sick and disoriented on the course, which is counterproductive. In addition, most people cannot roll in a straight line and will veer along the course, interfering with other racers. And, while this will vary from person to person, many of the obstacles are too low for people with wide shoulders. Lastly, many of the barbed-wire courses have rocks and other obstacles under the wire that you cannot see if you are rolling.

And a final word of advice here is, do not attempt to stand too early at the end of the obstacle as you will get caught in the barbs. Racers often assume that because their upper body is clear of the barbs, they can stand and move out. Always make sure that you are completely clear, including your legs, before attempting to stand up.

Tire Flip

The tire flip (see fig. 6.6) is an obstacle that can be very challenging if not done correctly. It will require you to flip a tire over a set distance or a specific number of times. There are three common methods that are used with this obstacle. It is very important to learn the proper technique so that you can successfully complete the task and significantly reduce the risk of injury.

The first method consists of three distinct movements: the drive, the catch, and the push. To begin, face the tire with your feet a little wider than shoulder-width apart and just in front of the tire. Place your arms close, just inside your legs, and squat down. Find a good grip under the tire with your arms bent, and lean into the tire, developing tension before the drive. Once in place, drive with your legs up and forward. Once you are fully extended, in one swift motion rotate your hands up and squat down, catching the tire. From this position, you will push the tire over.

The second option also has three phases: the drive, the step and knee, and the push. In this method, the drive occurs the same as before. The next step requires that you step forward with your left leg and drive your knee into the tire while rotating your hands up for the push. In the last phase, you push the tire over.

The last method is useful if the tires are too heavy or you become fatigued when required to conduct multiple flips. There are four stages here: the drive, the knee rest, reposition hands, and the march forward and push. As in the last two methods, the drive occurs in the same manner. Once you reach full extension on the drive, step forward with your right leg and let the tire rest on your leg. When you step forward, make sure that you keep your feet wide. Do not step forward in a manner that puts your right foot directly in front of your left foot as this position is very unstable. At this point, you can rest if you need to as the tire should be balanced. Next reposition your hands underneath as far as

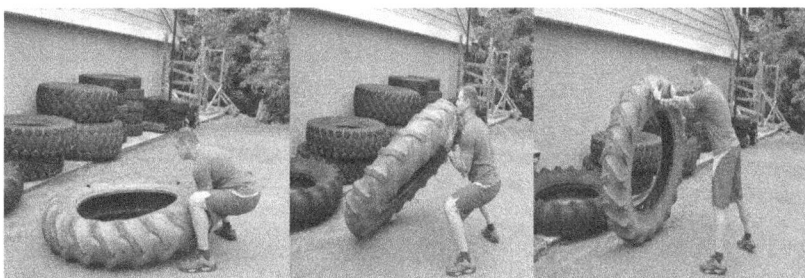

Figure 6.6. Tire flip. *Grayson Peveler.*

you can. Once your hands are in place, begin to march forward, bringing the tire upright, and then push it over.

Weighted Sled

The sled drag requires you to drag a weighted sled over a fixed distance. There are two basic variants to this obstacle. The first requires that you stay in place, grab the rope, and pull the sled toward you. The second involves you pulling the sled as you walk forward. I will discuss methods to use in both of these situations.

In the first scenario, the sled is attached to a long rope with the other end attached to a metal stake. You will be required to stand by the metal stake and pull the sled toward you until it reaches your position. Begin by squatting down, and then reach out and grab the rope with both hands. Extend your legs, dragging the sled toward you, and then squat down and repeat. While pulling with your arms helps, you want to primarily use your legs. Be careful not to lean too far back as you may fall backward if the sled moves suddenly.

Another option is to complete the sled pull in a seated position, similar to a seated row. To begin, sit down and plant your heels in the ground. Then grab the rope in both hands, using your legs and upper body to drag the sled toward you. Reset your position and repeat. You can also lean back to get more distance out of each pull. Be careful not to strain your back if you decide to lean back for extra distance.

A faster method is to place your feet a little wider than shoulder-width apart, grab the rope in both hands, and sit back with your legs slightly bent. Once you are set, begin pulling the rope toward you hand over hand. When you reach out and grab the rope, twist at the waist. When you pull back, rotate at the waist in the opposite direction. This motion engages your entire upper body as opposed to just using your arms. It takes a lot more force to start an object moving than it does to keep it moving. So, once you start, try not to stop. Although this is the fastest of the three methods, it is also the most fatiguing of the three due to primarily focusing on the use of your upper body.

Regardless of method, once the sled reaches your position at the stake, you must then drag it back into position for the next person. The handle used to drag it back is typically short, so you will have to walk backward as you drag it back into position.

The second common scenario requires you to move a weighted sled by walking forward over a fixed distance. This type of sled will have a long rope that creates a loop. The rope is long enough that you can step inside the loop and place it across your waist. Once you are in this position, lean forward and start driving with your legs, pulling the sled behind you. Again, it takes more force to start an object moving than it does to keep it moving, So once you start moving forward with the sled, try not to stop until you reach your destination.

Water Obstacles

Water obstacles can be both daunting and risky for those who are not comfortable in the water. So the first step to conquering water obstacles is to become comfortable both in the water and below the water's surface. There are no obstacles that require you to hold your breath for an extended period of time. However, work on breath holds and swimming underwater as the more comfortable you are, the easier the water obstacles will become. It is necessary to become a competent swimmer, which serves two purposes. The first is obvious, if a course requires swimming, you have it covered. The second is that as a competent swimmer, you will be more comfortable in the water in various situations.

Some obstacles require that you hold your breath, go under an obstacle, and come up on the other side. These obstacles are typically very thin, such as ½-inch plywood standing vertical. To make this obstacle much easier, place your arm under the obstacle and feel the other side. This will give you an idea of how far you have to go to reach the other side and may calm your nerves. With your other hand, grab the bottom of the obstacle to help guide you under. Take a deep breath and you will be on the other side in a couple seconds.

While not as frequent, you can run across obstacles that require you to travel through water in a confined space. Two of the most common obstacles here are submerged tunnels and flooded trenches. In the submerged tunnel obstacle, the tunnel is only partially filled with water, leaving plenty of room to move through the tunnel with your head above the water. The flooded trench has the top covered with metal fencing or a grate that can easily be pushed up if necessary. Lay on your back in the water and travel through the trench. There is plenty of room between the water and the grate to allow you to easily hold your head above the water as you move through. I usually like to make sure that the tunnel is clear prior to starting, in case someone freezes up.

At times you may have to travel along or across a creek or small river. When wading through the creek, pick your path carefully as you often cannot see the bottom. Feel for objects as you move your feet forward. Watch for changes in depth as you travel, and avoid deeper water when possible. Watch the people traveling in front of you so that you can judge the ease of travel and depth of the water prior to reaching that point. Stay away from algae-covered rocks as they are very slick and you can lose your footing quickly. Watch the current and make sure that you can handle it prior to entering.

Some obstacle races require jumping into the water from a height. When jumping into the water, never jump headfirst. Instead, always jump feetfirst as it is the safest way to enter the water. Before jumping, take the time to ensure that the area is clear of other racers. Landing on another racer can have devastating consequences for both of you.

When jumping, you want to hit the water straight up and down feetfirst. Keep your head centered over your center of mass in a straight line. The body will always follow the head. If your head is forward of your center of mass, you will begin to rotate forward as you fall. If your head is back, your body will rotate backward as you fall. Keep your legs straight and do not sit, in order to prevent your bottom and back of your legs from smacking the water. Hold your arms out to the side, in a nonrigid T shape, in order to maintain your balance in the air, and then pull them in tight and straight just prior to impact. Keep rigid during the entry, and then relax once you are submerged. Do not hold your nose as your arm will be ripped away from your face. Instead, exhale through your nose on impact.

The biggest mistake people make is to hesitate while jumping. If you watch failed jump attempts, you will notice that often jumpers hesitate or try to stop just as they jump, which results in a terrible water landing. Hesitation or trying to stop on takeoff results in you jumping off balance, making it impossible to determine how you will hit the water. Commit to the jump 100 percent, use good technique, and you will be fine.

SPECIAL
CONSIDERATIONS
FOR TRAINING AND
COMPETITION

Previous chapters discussed how the body responds and adapts to exercise, information that applies to everyone in general but may need to be modified based on factors such as age, gender, disease state, or disability. This chapter covers special considerations for specific populations that require adaptation to their training program in order to be successful: Due to gender differences, males and females respond slightly differently to training. As we age, the body alters and will not adapt to training in the same manner, and therefore training programs must adapt. Specific disease states alter the body's ability to adapt and may require special care and consideration. And finally, certain biomechanical and physiological adaptations must be made when working with disabled athletes as well.

WOMEN

In recent history female participation in sports has increased dramatically. When developing a training program for females, the same training principles discussed earlier can be applied without alterations. Women adapt to training stimuli in ways that are very similar to male athletes. However, there are some distinct differences, and there are a few key factors that should be taken into consideration when developing a training program.

Sex Differences

We should begin by acknowledging that there are key physiological differences between males and females. One of the primary differences involves hormones, primarily testosterone and estrogen. Males naturally produce 10 times more testosterone than females. Greater volumes of testosterone result in greater anabolic processes and therefore a significantly larger increase in muscle mass. Men can produce a faster contraction than women due to a greater speed of signaling, resulting in greater power. Muscle mass distribution also differs between males and females. A greater percentage of muscle mass is distributed in the upper body in males. It is important to note that there are no physiological differences between male and female muscle tissue and that the main difference in muscle mass is directly related to hormone levels. When looking at absolute strength, men are on average 30–60 percent stronger than females. These numbers are based on the average population. When looking at peer groups (racers of the same level and weight), the percentage differences are on the lower end. However, when you make the comparison based on weight lifted in relation to lean body mass, the differences decrease a little more.

Often women are concerned with becoming "bulky" or "looking like a guy" due to resistance training and therefore will avoid it. This is an unfounded concern as women do not produce the volume of testosterone that men do and therefore will not bulk up with resistance training designed for obstacle course racing. A female would have to develop a resistance training program designed to specifically bulk up in order to achieve that goal. Due to hormonal differences, it is much more difficult for females to put on muscle mass.

While females do not produce large amounts of testosterone, they do produce a large volume of estrogen, which affects the way females develop physiologically. One of the key roles of estrogen is increased lipid storage, particularly in the thighs and hips. This is the reason that essential body fat in females is 12 percent as opposed to 4 percent in males. Increased lipid storage is essential for the reproductive process. This is also why you can have a female racer and male racer of the same weight, yet the male is stronger because a greater percentage of his weight will be from lean muscle mass. Estrogen also plays an important part in female bone growth, as it increases calcium storage and retention.

Females also have a lower aerobic capacity in relation to their male counterparts. There are several factors that contribute to this phenomenon. The first is that males possess a larger overall blood volume and increased hemoglobin count per milliliter of blood compared to females. A greater hemoglobin count increases oxygen-carrying capacity, which in turn increases performance. To help offset lower levels of hemoglobin, females typically have higher levels of 2,3-DPG, which helps release oxygen into the tissue more easily. However, this does not completely compensate for the gender differences. Women also tend to have a smaller heart size, which in turn decreases stroke volume. All of these factors lead to a lower aerobic capacity, resulting in lower $VO_{2\,max}$ measures. At any given fitness level, females will produce $VO_{2\,max}$ scores that will be 5 to 10 ml/kg/min lower than their male counterparts.

While sex differences are scientifically verified, it does not mean that all males can outperform all females. The key is that males possess a higher aerobic capacity, greater lean muscle mass, and faster activation at any given level of competition. A pro female obstacle course racer could beat an amateur-level male racer; however, she would have difficulty with a pro male racer.

Female Athlete Triad

One of the common concerns for female athletes is the female athlete triad. As the name suggests, the triad consists of three distinct but interlocking components: inadequate caloric intake, amenorrhea, and osteoporosis. The process begins with inadequate caloric intake. Athletes expend a lot of calories, and when caloric expenditure consistently and excessively exceeds caloric intake, it creates a negative balance, resulting in an unhealthy body composition. As mentioned earlier, 12 percent body fat is considered essential in females. Those who drop below this percentage run the risk of developing the female athlete triad as well as other health discrepancies. This caloric imbalance is commonly brought on by the desire to optimize performance as well as concerns with body image.

Often the desire to optimize body composition for performance and body image can become an obsession and lead to eating disorders such as anorexia nervosa and bulimia. Over half of female athletes have been diagnosed with eating disorders. However, you do not have to have an eating disorder to be in a constant negative caloric balance. Training for OCR has a high caloric cost and therefore requires a high caloric intake. A female racer may appear to eat normally but still be in a negative caloric balance. When eating disorders are present, there is a strong psychological aversion to food or what food represents to that individual. In this case, the psychological aversion does not exist; they are just not eating adequately. It is a good idea to monitor caloric expenditure as well as caloric intake. Another way is to monitor body composition to ensure that you maintain essential body fat.

The next component of the female athlete triad is the development of abnormalities in the menstrual cycle, ultimately leading to amenorrhea (cessation of the menstrual cycle). Prolonged negative caloric balance and unhealthy body composition have a negative impact on the hypothalamus, reducing the release of gonadotropic hormones, which in turn impacts estrogen production and the menstrual cycle. An unhealthy body composition does not have to exist for amenorrhea to occur, however. High-intensity training has also been shown to lead to amenorrhea.

The final component of the female athlete triad is the development of osteoporosis, where bone density decreases, resulting in bones becoming brittle and easily fractured. Estrogen is responsible for the absorption and retention of calcium. When estrogen production greatly decreases with the cessation of the menstrual cycle, calcium absorption and retention greatly diminish, leading to a decrease in bone density. While the female athlete triad is a serious concern for women of all ages, special attention should be paid to those in their developmental years when bone growth is paramount.

Female Biomechanics

One of the main structural differences between males and females is the pelvic girdle. Women have a wider pelvic girdle and a wider sacrum, and the pelvis is shaped slightly differently. These differences are necessary to accommodate the birth process. These factors also lead to altered lower extremity biomechanics and a greater risk of lower extremity injuries compared to males. Knee injuries (primarily ACL ruptures) are more prevalent in female athletes. Female athletes are six to eight times more likely to rupture an ACL than male athletes of the same sport. Knee injuries, including ACL ruptures, are quite common in obstacle course racing. One method for decreasing the risk of injury is to strengthen the knee extensors (quadriceps) and the knee flexors (hamstrings). Typically, the quadriceps muscles will be significantly stronger than the hamstring muscles. Research supports that the less there is of a strength difference between the extensors and flexors, the less likely an injury will occur.

Pregnancy

Research has demonstrated that there are many benefits for women who exercise during pregnancy. Some of the proposed benefits are a decrease in excessive weight gain, decreased labor pains, a decreased risk of developing gestational diabetes, and an easier return to pre-pregnancy weight and fitness level after birth. Exercise during pregnancy should only be conducted by women who are experiencing a normal pregnancy and have their doctor's permission.

Remember, only your doctor can determine if you are healthy enough to exercise and at what level you can train.

If you become pregnant, sit down and have an honest and detailed conversation with your doctor concerning exercise. When it has been established that you are experiencing a normal, healthy pregnancy, then discuss your goals and training plan with your doctor. The doctor will establish your training limitations, which you should follow precisely. Throughout the pregnancy, continue to maintain an open dialogue regarding your training.

When pregnant, training goals should be altered. You should eliminate risk of impact from your training. As pregnancy progresses, balance becomes compromised: as the baby grows and the belly protrudes, the body's center of gravity shifts. At this point, eliminate obstacles from your training, but other forms of training will still be possible, assuming you have your doctor's clearance to do so.

During pregnancy, a hormone, relaxin, is released in order to relax the pelvis to prepare for birth. Unfortunately, relaxin also causes other joints in the lower extremities to loosen too, which leads to decreased stability and balance.

Training intensity will also need to be lowered. Blood flow is redirected during exercise to the working muscles and to the skin for cooling, which in turn reduces blood flow to the fetus. At mild to moderate intensity, reduced blood flow does not impact fetus health. However, as intensity increases, a greater amount of blood is redirected from the uterus. It is for this reason that vigorous high-intensity exercise should be avoided during pregnancy. When training, it is okay to exercise until you feel slightly fatigued, but never exercise to exhaustion while pregnant. Due to alterations in blood flow during pregnancy, heart rate becomes an unreliable tool for determining exercise intensity. Instead, use perceived exertion to determine intensity.

Due to reduced blood flow to the skin and increased insulation, your ability to dissipate heat is greatly compromised during pregnancy. A significant increase in the fetus's core temperature can negatively impact development. Do not train in the heat, stay well hydrated, and be mindful of any significant increase in core temperature. Train during a cooler part of the day or inside to avoid overheating.

Exercising in a supine position, on your back, is also not recommended during pregnancy, as it lowers cardiac output and can restrict blood flow to the fetus. Find alternate exercises to replace those that you typically conduct in a supine position.

AGING

Aging has a strong impact on our ability to adapt to training. We are all on a theoretical curve where physical abilities increase through life until they peak somewhere between the ages of 25 and 30 years old. We can briefly maintain that peak until our physical abilities begin to gradually decline around the ages of about 35 to 40. This curve remains true for all healthy individuals. Naturally, someone who trains will have a higher performance level at any point in the curve when compared to a sedentary individual.

Fitness level along this curve can be altered by increasing or decreasing physical activity. If a collegiate athlete who has been active his entire life stopped training after college, his fitness level would drop down to the level of someone who is sedentary. The reverse is true for someone who has been sedentary his whole life and then decides to start training. However, the basic principle still remains true in that your ability to adapt to training will begin to diminish around the age of 35 with a significant decline starting around 45 years of age.

Aerobic capacity also decreases significantly with age. It is estimated that there is a reduction in $VO_{2\,max}$ of approximately 1 ml/kg/min a year. Much of the age-related decrease in $VO_{2\,max}$ is due to a significant reduction in physical activity, which occurs as an individual ages. Those who remain active throughout life can offset the loss in $VO_{2\,max}$. While not as steep a decline, those who remain active will still see a reduction in aerobic capacity due to a reduction in cardiovascular function and an age-related decrease in muscle mass (sarcopenia).

Sarcopenia is a common component of aging. However, the extent of the decline in muscle mass is highly dependent on the individual's fitness level. For those who remain active throughout life, the decrease is lessened. While physical activity goes a long way toward preventing loss of muscle mass, it cannot completely offset sarcopenia. The aging process results in a large decrease in hormone production, resulting in a decrease in protein synthesis and, therefore, a decrease in muscle mass.

With age there is a naturally occurring decrease in bone density. There are two distinct stages: osteopenia and osteoporosis. Osteopenia is a decrease in bone density that occurs prior to the development of osteoporosis and is much less severe. Bones at this stage are more susceptible to damage compared to normal bone, but less susceptible in relation to bones in an osteoporotic state. Osteoperosis is a severe decrease in bone density, resulting in a greater susceptibility to fractures. Both states occur due to age-related decreases in hormones. In males there is a link between an age-related decrease in testosterone production and a decrease in bone density. In females there is a strong relationship between estrogen levels and bone density. This leaves postmenopausal women strongly susceptible to the development of osteoporosis due to a significant decrease in estrogen production. Estrogen is a key hormone in the absorption and retention of calcium in females. Since estrogen production is greatly diminished with age, the absorption and retention of calcium decreases, leading to a reduction of bone density.

There are two main things that you can do to help prevent a decrease in bone density. First, consistently maintain a healthy, well-balanced diet. Second, participate in weight-bearing activities. Bones respond to stress in the same basic manner that muscles do. If you apply adequate mechanical stress to the bone, then bone density increases. If inadequate mechanical stress is applied to bone, then bone density decreases. Weight-bearing activity is the only way to increase bone density. Examples of weight-bearing activities are running, lifting, plyometrics, and heavy bag workouts. Running is a weight-bearing activity that can lead to increased bone density. However, the mechanical stress is focused on the lower body and does nothing to increase bone density in the upper body. Therefore, when developing a program with bone density in mind, it is important to choose activities that will apply a mechanical load for the entire body. Resistance training is weight bearing and allows for adequate stress to be applied to almost all bones in the body. Resistance exercises conducted when training for obstacle course racing are excellent for increasing bone density as they are weight-bearing activities.

These recommendations are not guaranteed protection against the development of osteopenia and osteoporosis, however. There is also a genetic component for the development of these disorders. But maintaining a proper diet and including weight-bearing activities in your training are vital steps toward maintaining proper bone density. Keep in mind that obstacle course racing places a large amount of stress on bone, and therefore it is very important to maintain bone density in order to offset the risk of fractures due to training and competition.

A significant a decrease in cardiac output occurs with aging. This decrease is a result of a diminished stroke volume and maximal heart rate. The age-related decrease in stroke volume occurs due to a reduction in the left ventricle's ability to expand and contract, resulting in less blood ejected from the heart each beat. At the same time, there is an estimated decrease in maximal heart rate by one beat per minute (bpm) each year. The decrease in maximal heart rate is believed to be attributed to age-related changes to the cardiac-conduction system (electrical signaling for contraction) combined with decreased sensitivity of the myocardium to specific hormones, primarily epinephrine and norepinephrine.

A decrease in cardiac output results in a corresponding decrease in aerobic performance.

Another key factor in an age-related decline in performance is the lessened ability to recover between training bouts, resulting in a decrease in an individual's ability to handle higher volumes and intensities. Monitor your response to training as you age, and adapt the training program accordingly. There will come a point when both intensity and volume will need to be adjusted to allow time for adequate recovery. The exact timing is variable and will be highly dependent on your age, training status, health, and training goals.

There is a decrease in neuromuscular response as you age. You will notice diminished performance in reaction times, neuromuscular recruitment patterns, and speed of contraction. The greatest impact is seen in voluntary muscle responses to a stimulus. An example would be a decrease in your ability to make a quick adjustment when slipping on an overhead obstacle. Staying physically active will offset this decline, but it will not completely negate it.

Flexibility also decreases as we age. There are various reasons for this, for example, problems at the joints, decrease in elasticity of the muscle, etc. But the primary reason for such a decrease is directly related to a lack of flexibility training. If you want to stay flexible as you age, maintain a flexibility program.

Do not let age-related decreases in performance discourage you from pursuing your goal. Use this information to help develop a training program that will optimize your increases in performance. Keep in mind that increases in performance can occur at any age and therefore should not hinder anyone from starting a program. It is important to note that fitness gains for someone beginning a training program at age 45 will not occur as quickly or be as large as an individual who started a program at 20, assuming both are utilizing the same program. Training can lead to increases in muscle mass, decreases in body fat, increases in bone density, and lower blood pressure, and can positively impact cholesterol levels and provide many other health benefits. While medical clearance is important for all ages, it is vitally important that older individuals consult a physician prior to beginning an exercise program.

CHILDREN AND ADOLESCENTS

For the purpose of this section, childhood is defined as age 6 to puberty, and adolescence is defined as the time period from puberty to 18 years of age. Getting our youth involved in physical activity at an early age is extremely important, and OCR is an excellent way to do it.

Children and adolescents differ from adults both physiologically and psychologically. It is important to understand these differences as children should not be trained as small adults. The main physiological difference involves hormone levels. Prior to puberty, children produce very small amounts of hormones and therefore cannot adapt to training as effectively as adults. Research has demonstrated that performance gains in prepubescent children occur in areas of aerobic performance, anaerobic performance, muscular endurance, and muscular strength. However, the mechanisms behind these improvements occur through physiological pathways that are slightly, but importantly, different than adults.

With endurance training, children can experience significant gains in aerobic performance. However, with these gains there is little to no change in their aerobic capacity or $VO_{2\,max}$ measurements. Instead, increases in aerobic performance are attributed to improved neuromuscular recruitment patterns. As the child's technique improves, he becomes more economical and his aerobic performance improves dramatically with no alteration to aerobic capacity.

This same basic concept applies to resistance training as well. With resistance training children can see an increase in both muscular strength and muscular endurance. This increase in strength is not due to muscle hypertrophy, but instead occurs due to neuromuscular adaptations that occur through training. Children under the age of 13 should only be doing bodily muscular endurance resistance training and should not be lifting heavy weight.

The overall key message is that training for children should not focus on attempting to alter aerobic capacity or strength. Instead the training programs should focus on producing proper technique, leading to optimizing recruitment patterns.

Training for kids should focus on having fun while learning. At this stage, training should not feel like a chore, and children should look forward to it. The biggest mistake people make here is forcing training on children and working them too hard. Watch and listen to your child, and she will let you know when she is tired and needs a break.

During puberty, hormone levels begin to increase. As a child reaches adolescence, the ability to adapt to training, beyond just neuromuscular, improves dramatically. During puberty, male testosterone production increases to about 10 times that of prepubescent levels, resulting in a substantially increased rate of growth. During this period, joints may not be as stable, which may result in pain and possible injury during sports. Once puberty is reached, both volume and intensity can increase, but not yet to the level of an adult. An adolescent can begin an entry-level adult program at the age of 16. This is an average age, and programs should be individualized as some adolescents mature faster or slower than others.

Another aspect to consider when working with youth is that they are still developing psychologically. Children and adolescents may not be able to readily grasp complicated concepts. So keep the explanations simple and expressed in terms they can understand. This will not only get the concept across to them but will also prevent them from becoming frustrated.

Avoid training intensities and training volumes that are too high. In recent history, sports-related injuries have drastically increased in children due to improper training volumes. Children are developing overuse injuries that typically do not occur in athletes until their collegiate or professional careers. One of the primary reasons for this is that adult training programs are being applied to children and adolescents. Another reason is that kids are now playing sports at a high volume and intensity year-round. It is highly recommended that children stay active year-round, however, and OCR is an excellent way to stay active. But it is important to keep track of the overall training volume and intensity to prevent overtraining and overuse injuries. Not every training session needs to be high intensity. It is also important to account for your child's other sports when considering overall training load.

WEIGHT AND OBESITY

Obstacle course racing is an excellent way to improve health and lose weight, and many become involved in the sport for this reason. Research shows that individuals who are overweight and physically active are significantly less likely to develop cardiovascular disease than thin, inactive people. You do not have to look like one of the people on the front of a magazine to be healthy. There are certain key points you should consider when training for obstacle course racing while overweight or obese, however.

If you are overweight, you are much more susceptible to the development of heat-related injuries as fat storage acts as insulation, reducing the body's ability to effectively dissipate heat. While this can be beneficial on cold days, it is counterproductive on hot, humid days. When training in the heat, be cognizant of signs and symptoms of heat-related illness.

Running is a weight-bearing activity and the impact (ground reaction forces) are two to three times your body weight. Due to the impact of running, begin training slowly, listen to your body, and make adjustments accordingly. Starting your running program at too high a volume or intensity may result in the development of overuse injuries, such as stress fractures or joint injuries. It is normal to feel slight discomfort, but you should not feel pain during a run. The development of sharp pains is a sign of possible damage and should be evaluated by a physician. You may even want to begin your aerobic program with activities that are non–weight bearing, such as cycling. This will give you the aerobic improvements without undue stress on the joints. You can add running to your program as you progress.

DIABETES

Diagnosed diabetics are typically well versed on their disease, treatment, and symptoms. While you may be confident that you can manage your diabetes, you should still consult with your doctor when beginning a training program for obstacle course racing. This section is not intended to provide medical advice, but instead to discuss a few key considerations that you may wish to discuss with your doctor. When developing a plan with your doctor, discuss how to alter diet and insulin injections, if needed, to accommodate your current level of training.

Another reason for obtaining a physician's clearance prior to starting a training program is that diabetes can result in the development of other health complications. Some of the common comorbidities are high blood pressure, cardiovascular disease, compromised peripheral vascularization, and peripheral neuropathy. While exercise is recommended for individuals with diabetes, it is important that diabetes is under control prior to starting a program and that control is maintained throughout training. Once cleared to participate in physical activity, you must monitor blood glucose levels before, during, and after training and adjust accordingly.

Diabetics are also well versed in the pathophysiology of the disease and its related factors. The following information is more for the coaches and trainers who may be working with diabetics. While there are other pathologies, I will discuss the two basic pathologies for the occurrence of diabetes. The first occurs when the insulin-producing cells located on the pancreas are damaged, which ultimately limits insulin production. This is usually due to an autoimmune dysfunction where the body's immune system attacks the cells. Because the pancreas cannot produce adequate amounts of insulin, many diabetics will need to inject insulin into their system. This type of diabetes is typically referred to as type I or early onset diabetes.

Whereas type I diabetes is a result of a decrease in insulin production, type II diabetes is a result of a decrease in insulin sensitivity at the insulin receptor sites.

Insulin receptor sites are down regulated (reduction in hormone receptor sites) in response to chronic high levels of insulin being released into the system. This commonly occurs due to consumption of an overabundance of foods that are high on the glycemic index, resulting in regular insulin spikes in order to offset spikes in blood glucose. However, the two primary risk factors for the development of type II diabetes are being sedentary and being overweight.

Both exercise and proper diet have a strong effect on both type I and type II diabetes. Due to the permanent damage to the islet beta cells of the pancreas, exercise and proper diet do not provide a cure for type I diabetes. However, a combination of exercise and diet can positively impact it by helping keep the disease under better control. Diet and exercise have a much stronger impact on type II diabetes as they increase insulin sensitivity.

If you have diabetes, work with a registered dietitian who is familiar with sport performance. It is unlikely that the average coach would have sufficient knowledge to adequately assess and prescribe proper nutrition to a diabetic, and some state regulations even prohibit giving nutritional advice to those with a disease state such as diabetes.

Low blood sugar (hypoglycemia) is of great concern for diabetic athletes, which is why it is important to monitor blood glucose levels before, during, and after exercise. Glycogen (the storage form of blood sugar) and glucose are the only sources of energy the brain can utilize. Therefore, when blood glucose levels are low, the brain and central nervous systems are negatively impacted. The initial response to low blood sugar is the release of epinephrine (commonly referred to as adrenaline) in an attempt to increase blood sugar. The release of epinephrine results in a significant increase in heart rate, the development of muscle tremors, anxiety, and an increased appetite. These are the most common early warning symptoms of hypoglycemia. As hypoglycemia begins to affect the brain, symptoms worsen, resulting in headache, dizziness, fatigue, irritability, slurred speech, blurred vision, confusion, lack of coordination, and unconsciousness. In severe cases hypoglycemia can even result in coma or death.

Hypoglycemia can progress very quickly, and training should cease instantly upon presentation of symptoms. The athlete should then immediately measure blood glucose and respond accordingly. Diabetic athletes will typically keep foods high on the glycemic index available to help counteract a hypoglycemic episode. The athlete should eat, recheck blood sugar levels, and then make an educated decision on whether or not to continue training. If blood sugar levels are not within the normal limits or the athlete does not feel well, the training session should be canceled.

Training for OCR places a heavy strain on glycogen stores and blood glucose levels, and therefore adjustments to both diet and insulin may need to be considered. It is important to remember that blood glucose is released from the liver and into the blood at a much higher rate during anaerobic bouts. Insulin-dependent racers may need to adjust insulin timing and dosage. Diabetic racers who use an insulin pump should take this into consideration when training and competing as there is risk of the insertion site becoming loose or infected. Often when competing in an obstacle course race, you will traverse stagnant water, which will increase the risk of infection at the insertion site. Pumps may not be waterproof and could easily be damaged on an obstacle. Often racers who use a pump switch to shots on the day of the race. This is not medical advice, and I am just stating that these are common concerns. It is very important that you not make any alteration to your diet or timing, delivery system, and dosage of insulin before thoroughly discussing it with your physician prior to implementation.

ASTHMA

Asthma is characterized by difficulty breathing and is one of the most common chronic diseases that affects athletes. During an asthma attack, the air passage constricts and mucus builds up, interfering with normal breathing. The severity of asthma attacks varies and ranges from slight discomfort while breathing to a life-threatening blockage. For some athletes, asthma only occurs in relation to physical exertion, where an episode will occur only during or shortly after exercise, and is known as exercise-induced asthma. It is important to note that asthmatic symptoms can present 5 to 10 minutes after the cessation of exercise. Any asthma trigger (pollen, carbon monoxide, etc.) can increase the risk of exercise-induced asthma. Environmental factors also play a role. Cold, dry environments greatly increase the risk of an incident, whereas warm, humid environments reduce the risk.

A slow, gradual, and longer warm-up is recommended for those diagnosed with asthma. If you have frequent or severe asthma, pay close attention to your warm-up protocol. If prescribed by a physician, an inhaler can be used prior to competition in order to help prevent an occurrence. Never train without your inhaler physically present. As a coach it is always a good idea to have the athlete show their inhaler prior to the start of any session. Inhalers contain banned substances (primarily albuterol), and therefore use of an inhaler requires a medical waiver.

PHYSICAL DISABILITIES

I believe that participating in obstacle course racing is an excellent idea for everyone, and I do not believe that disabilities should discourage or eliminate anyone from racing. For the context of this discussion, "disabilities" will be an all-encompassing term, covering everything from physical, intellectual, and neuromuscular diseases. Running biomechanics, techniques for traversing obstacles, and strength-and-conditioning techniques can be adapted to accommodate an athlete's individual disability. You can find numerous examples of disabled athletes who have been very successful competing in obstacle course racing. It is beyond the scope of this section to give detailed advice for specific disabilities, so instead I will focus on general advice.

The first important step is to know and understand your specific disability as it relates to physical activity. Adjustments in technique may be required. Do not get stuck in the trap of trying to precisely follow the taught techniques when your disability prevents you from doing so. It will be frustrating and nonproductive. Instead, focus on the idea of the technique and what that technique is supposed to accomplish. Once you understand the desired outcome, the next step is to develop a technique to accommodate for your disability that produces the same desired outcome. This is true for any physical activity, whether it be obstacle technique, lifting, or running.

There is not a sport that does not have a related risk of injury. Some sports do possess greater risk than others, and there is risk involved when competing in obstacle course racing. Depending on your disability, you may or may not be at greater risk than the average athlete. Therefore, it is important to understand your specific disability-related risks when it comes to participating in obstacle course racing. Speak with your doctor about your desire to become involved in obstacle course racing, and discuss any specific concerns for participation, increased risks of participation, and adaptations that need to be made in order for you to safely and effectively participate. After speaking with your doctor, make a list of all concerns, risks, and necessary adaptations, and develop a strong training and racing plan.

If you have a coach, educate your coach about your disability. They may have never coached an athlete with your specific disability before, and the more knowledge they have, the better they can assist you in reaching your goals. It is not only important to educate them about your specific disability but also to let them know you are not made of glass and that you are there to participate to the fullest of your ability and want to be challenged, to learn, and to grow just like anyone else they coach.

Lastly, there are many organizations that work with disabled athletes. The International Paralympic Committee is a great resource for disabled athletes (https://www.paralympic.org/). While obstacle course racing is not currently a Paralympic sport, they do include related sports, such as running. And all athletes will have a strength-and-conditioning program. There are many other organizations that provide training and information for disabled athletes. These organizations not only provide information but also provide an opportunity for you to connect with other athletes who have similar disabilities and are willing to share their experiences. Reach out and find an organization that fits best with your personal situation.

8

INJURY AND INJURY PREVENTION

This chapter is designed to provide basic information on injury and injury prevention. Obstacle course racing is a moderate-risk sport, and injuries are not uncommon in both training and competition. This chapter will focus on injuries where preventable measures exist. I will discuss both the mechanism of the injury and any possible injury-prevention strategies. Muscular sprains, muscular tears, joint damage, and fractures occurring in an obstacle course race are a real possibility. However, all those injuries require medical attention and are beyond the scope of this book. The following is not meant to be medical advice, and you should always be evaluated by a doctor when any injury occurs.

PHYSICAL EXAM

Prior to beginning an OCR program, it is important that you get a physical exam to ensure that you are healthy enough to participate. If you have been inactive up to this point, it is even more important to have a physical exam prior to starting, as being sedentary is a major risk factor for the development of cardiovascular disease, type II diabetes, high cholesterol, high blood pressure, and other medical problems. A physical exam may discover medical conditions that you may not be aware you have.

If you have a diagnosed disease state, doctors will often recommend physical activity as a method for improving overall health. If you are currently being treated for a specific disease state, it is important that you consult with your doctor prior to participating in obstacle course racing. Your doctor will be in the best position to advise you on your involvement in the sport.

It is recommended that older individuals (males over age 45 and females over 55) seek medical clearance prior to beginning any exercise program. As we age, we become more susceptible to the development of specific disease states, such as cardiovascular disease. As OCR can place a heavy demand on your cardiovascular system, it is vital that older individuals, and anyone showing signs or symptoms of cardiovascular disease, obtain medical clearance prior to beginning.

Below is a list of the common signs and symptoms associated with cardio-vascular disease. The following list is not all inclusive and these symptoms only indicate the possibility of the disease. Only your physician can diagnose it or rule it out. Also, keep in mind that cardiovascular disease can be asymptomatic.

- chest pain at rest or during exercise
- pain in the arms, shoulder, neck, or jaw region
- abnormal shortness of breath
- irregular heartbeat (speed or rhythm)
- edema in the ankles
- cramping in the calf muscles
- unusual fatigue
- dizziness
- fainting
- difficulty breathing when lying down

When looking for a primary physician, I always recommend finding a sports-specific doctor or at least a physician who understands athletes. They will have a better understanding of the stress you will be putting your body through, how the body responds to training, and the mind-set that goes along with being an athlete.

When suffering from muscular injuries, connective tissue damage, or bone damage, I recommend seeking medical advice from an orthopedic sports-medicine specialist. These practitioners have a strong background in sports medicine, giving them insight into the mechanisms behind the injury and what it will take to optimally get you back to training and competing. They can make better decisions on your training load and what you can and cannot currently handle given your specific situation.

ILLNESS

Overall, exercise is good for the body and results in improved immune function in healthy individuals. However, a hard training session actually challenges the immune system, making you more susceptible to developing an illness just after completion of training. In addition, athletes who are frequently overtrained often develop compromised immune function. Frequent or persistent illness is a common sign of overtraining.

There are a few general guidelines to follow for training when ill. In most cases, training should be avoided when you do not feel well as your illness may become worse or last longer than it would have otherwise. Training should be avoided if you feel nauseous, have a fever, a headache, or body aches, or are experiencing severe fatigue. In most cases, you are okay to train with a cold as long as you do not have a fever or body aches and you have no chest congestion.

When your immune system is already fighting an illness, training will further suppress it. Missing a few days of training to recover from an illness will not completely derail your training program, whereas, attempting to push through an illness could make it worse and result in increased time off from training.

When taking over-the-counter or prescribed medication, know how it can interact with exercise. For example, decongestants can act as a stimulant, resulting in a significant increase in resting and submaximal heart rates. While this may not be harmful, it can result in alteration to training zones while on decongestants. Decongestants can also cause dehydration and drowsiness. Always ask your doctor about the interactions of your medication and exercise.

URINARY TRACT INFECTIONS

Urinary tract infections (UTI) are a common problem for females and even more so in female athletes. A urinary tract infection occurs when bacteria enters the urethra and travels to the bladder. There are two common areas where you may experience greater than normal bacteria in an obstacle course race. The first is in your running shorts. As you exercise, your body temperature increases and you sweat. Your shorts become wet, providing an excellent breeding ground for bacteria. The second area will be in any water obstacles you must traverse. To decrease the risk of developing a UTI after a race, remove your shorts, urinate, and shower as soon as possible after competition.

GASTROINTESTINAL ISSUES

It is quite common to encounter muddy, stagnant water when participating in an obstacle course race. This water and mud can contain bacteria (such as C. coli) and parasites (such as giardia) that can easily enter the system by swallowing the contaminated water or mud, resulting in gastrointestinal distress. Some of these races are held in fields with cattle, pigs, and other animals in close proximity. The nearby feces contain bacteria and parasites. This greatly increases the risk of possible infection.

Bacteria can easily enter the system through open wounds or the eyes, nose, and mouth. However, for this section, we will focus on bacteria entering only through the nose or mouth. Bacterial infections and open wounds will be discussed below.

Bacterial infections result in diarrhea, abdominal pain, nausea, and fever. The symptoms can appear up to five days after the race. However, typically the symptoms present within a few days. Often symptoms alleviate fairly quickly without intervention, but it is not uncommon to require medical assistance. If your illness is severe or persistent, or if you are in doubt, seek medical attention.

On the surface, symptoms of giardiasis are the same as a bacterial infection, making it very difficult to distinguish between the two. The symptoms for giardiasis usually begin 7 to 21 days after the race. If giardiasis is suspected, seek medical treatment.

To prevent infection, attempt to keep your face clear of water and mud as much as possible and avoid swallowing any water. While it is an obstacle race and your face will get muddy and wet, avoid unnecessary contact. If you have a hydration pack, attempt to keep the mouthpiece as clean as possible throughout the race. Once the race is finished, clean up thoroughly. Do not attempt to eat anything prior to cleaning up as bacteria or parasites on your hands and face can enter the system when eating.

ABRASIONS

Abrasions are quite common when competing in obstacle course racing. They typically occur when traversing an obstacle or from falling on the course. Skin abrasions occur as your skin travels across a surface, creating friction burns and lacerations. Abrasions are open wounds and should be treated as such. If the abrasion is serious, seek medical attention immediately. If lacerations are present, those should be addressed by a doctor as well. In most cases, abrasions are small enough to address at home. When sliding across the trail, small rocks, dirt, and other debris can become embedded in the wound and will need to be cleaned out in order to decrease the risk of infection. Make sure to clean the wound of all debris with a medical scrub brush. After the wound has been cleaned, coat it with ointment. Depending on the location and seriousness of the wound, you can keep it covered during the oozing stage.

As mentioned previously, in obstacle course racing bacterial infections are not uncommon due to moving through stagnant, muddy water, an excellent breeding ground for bacteria. When open wounds are submerged where bacteria thrive, infections can occur. To help prevent infections, make sure to thoroughly clean all open wounds. As wounds heal watch for signs of infection. Common signs of infection are listed below:

- swelling
- increased pain
- wound enlarging
- spreading redness around the wound
- fever
- puss and drainage

BLISTERS

This section will focus on friction blisters that can occur on the hands and feet due to friction between your skin and another object. The movement between your skin and the object causes the skin to separate and then fill with fluid, leaving a blister. Blisters will most likely occur in the hands from climbing obstacles, overhead obstacles, and rope obstacles. Blisters that occur on the feet will most likely be from running. Treatment for most blisters is simple: leave them alone. It is important not to pick the skin off the top of a blister and to just let it heal. If the skin does come off, treat it as an open wound. As with any wound, watch for signs of infection.

Through training you will develop calluses on your hands and fingers, which naturally help prevent the formation of blisters. You can use gloves during obstacles in order to provide a layer of protection as well. I am not personally a fan of gloves because I like to feel the obstacles for better control. Other people swear by gloves. Decide what works best for you.

Blisters on the feet and toes are a common problem with many racers. There are some key steps you can take to help reduce the risk of developing blisters. The first is to make sure that you are running in the correct shoes and that those shoes fit properly. Do not race in shoes that are not designed for the task or that do not fit well. Another big mistake is buying a new pair of shoes for the race and then racing without ever training in them. Socks that are too thin, do not wick moisture away, or bunch up are another common reason for blisters, so be sure that you are running in a good pair of socks. Some individuals are more susceptible to blisters than others. If your shoes and socks are good, the next step is to protect the areas where you commonly get blisters. You can cover the area with medical tape to add a layer of protection. You will need to practice with this method prior to racing as it may be tricky to get the tape to stay in place without bunching up. Another option is to apply liquid bandage to the areas where you commonly blister. If you choose this method, you will want to apply the liquid bandage the night before the race and not just prior. This gives it plenty of time to dry so you can determine if you need another coat the next morning.

ANTERIOR CRUCIATE LIGAMENT

The anterior cruciate ligament (ACL) is attached to the femur and tibia and is used to provide anterior stability to the knee. The ACL is commonly injured during contact sports and sports that have strong cutting motions. During obstacle course racing there are two primary mechanisms that commonly result in ACL tears. The first involves planting the foot and then abruptly changing direction. The second involves landing from a high jump. Anterior cruciate ligament tears can put you out of commission for an extended period of time for surgery and recovery. Gender also is a factor as females are six to eight times more likely to develop an ACL injury than their male counterparts due to biomechanical gender differences.

There are a few methods you can utilize to reduce the risk of ACL injury. The first is to work on strengthening muscles of the lower extremities. The stronger the joint, the less likely it will subluxate or dislocate. The second is to offset any strength discrepancies between the quadriceps and hamstrings. It is common for the quadricep muscles to be significantly stronger than the hamstring muscles. This causes a greater anterior pull on the knee and greater stress on the anterior cruciate ligament. Increasing the strength of the hamstring muscles offsets this discrepancy and increases the stability of the knee. Improving agility and balance will also assist in dynamic knee stability. Learning to land properly from a ground jump or when jumping from a height is also important. While none of these procedures will completely eliminate the risk of an ACL injury, they will significantly reduce it.

OVERUSE INJURIES

Unfortunately, overuse injuries are quite common when training for obstacle course racing. OCR requires repetitive motions that place stress on the muscles, connective tissues, bones, and joint structures. An overuse injury presents as chronic pain in a specific area that is directly related to training. An overuse injury can hurt before, during, and after training. Some overuse injuries may feel fine during training but then hurt after training or the next day when getting out of bed (plantar fasciitis is an example). The pain can range from mild and annoying to excruciating. If not addressed appropriately, the damage and pain can increase with continued training. Persistent pain should be evaluated by a doctor.

There are many factors that can attribute to overuse injuries. Many of these factors relate to improper training. One of the common mistakes made by beginning racers is increasing training volume or intensity too quickly. Remember to progress your training in a controlled and correctly paced manner. Always increase your volume first and then increase your intensity once you establish a solid base.

Another common cause of overuse injury is overtraining. It is important to allow adequate recovery time between training bouts. When you ignore necessary recovery time, it leaves the body in a weakened state that is susceptible to the development of an overuse injury. Be as diligent about your recovery as you are about your training.

Lack of flexibility is another leading cause of overuse injuries. I cannot count the number of athletes I have worked with whose overuse injury was the result of lack of flexibility. Once the flexibility issues were addressed, the overuse injury subsided. When joints are not able to easily go through their full range of motion during exercise, it can result in undue strain in that area and the development of an overuse injury.

Muscular strength around a joint can also play a factor in the development of overuse injuries. The weaker the muscles around a joint, the less stable that joint is and the more susceptible to the development of an overuse injury. Muscular imbalances can also lead to the development of an overuse injury. For example, if the quadriceps muscles are significantly stronger than the hamstring muscles, it will result in an anterior pull at the knee, resulting in static and dynamic instability. The closer the match in strength between the hamstring and quadriceps muscles, the more stable the joint will be. Not only should you work on increasing strength but also on ensuring muscular balance.

And finally, improper biomechanics or technique can lead to the development of an overuse injury even when all other factors are accounted for.

Lower Body

Running is a consistent activity throughout an obstacle course race. This activity applies a large amount of force to the lower body. Every time the foot strikes the ground, the ground reaction force is two to three times the body mass of the runner. If you are running an eight-minute-per-mile pace with an average cadence of 170 steps per minute for a five-mile run, then you will strike the ground approximately 6,800 times at two to three times your body mass.

Overuse injuries can occur when running as a result of biomechanical insufficiencies. When running, the ground reaction force travels up the kinetic chain from ground contact. Biomechanical abnormalities result in improper transfer of energy up the chain. It is important to identify and address any biomechanical insufficiency that may exist. The most common overuse injuries that occur due to running and jumping are:

Shin Splints

Shin splints are not uncommon in runners and present as pain in the lower anterior portion of the leg as a result of damage to the soft tissue (primarily connective tissue). When volume or intensity are increased too quickly, especially in beginning runners, shin splints may occur. Running in shoes that are worn out, do not fit properly, or are not meant for running are also common causes. Shin splints can also occur due to biomechanical abnormalities, such as severe overpronation, joint instability, or lack of flexibility. If you have persistent shin splints, you may want to see a doctor as it could be something more serious such as stress fractures or compartment syndrome.

Knee Pain

Knee pain in runners is often referred to as "runner's knee." Frequently, runners use this term as a catchall for any pain that occurs in the area of the knee while running. By this definition, there are numerous issues that could be occurring. When medical professionals discuss runner's knee, it is specific to the anterior portion of the knee centered around the patella. There are two common pathologies for this. The first involves pain centered directly behind the patella. This pain is most often a result of improper tracking of the patella and undue pressure on the patella as it passes across the femur. This scenario can result in the development of chondromalacia (deterioration of cartilage on the posterior patella). The second common pathology is pain along the patellar tendon (patella tendonitis). Common causes of runner's knee are muscular weaknesses, muscular imbalances, patella tracking issues, and repetitive strain placed on the knee while running.

Constant knee pain should be evaluated by a doctor to ensure that you are not causing greater damage by continuing to run. There are a few steps you can take to help alleviate the problem. The first is to ensure that you are running in good running shoes that fit correctly. Another is to strengthen the muscles around the joint in order to increase stability of the joint area and to possibly help with any patella tracking issues. Increase your flexibility so that you can comfortably go through the full range of motion at each joint. Pay close attention to the hamstrings and glutes as this is where most runners are tight.

Plantar Fasciitis

Plantar fasciitis presents as pain along the bottom of the foot located at the heel. Plantar fasciitis can be very painful. The plantar fascia is the connective tissue that runs along the bottom of the foot from the calcaneus of the heel to the toes and is responsible for maintaining the longitudinal arch of the foot. Plantar fasciitis occurs when the plantar fascia becomes damaged and inflamed. While damage can occur acutely, it often occurs due to repeated stress. The pain is felt when running, but it can worsen after a run. Plantar fasciitis can be very painful when getting out of bed in the morning or if you have been in a stationary period for a prolonged period of time, such as sitting at a desk. This soreness occurs due to the plantar fascia shortening and tightening. It is not uncommon for the pain to decrease throughout the day when the fascia loosens up as you move around. It is often recommended to sleep in a night splint as it keeps the foot in a neutral position and keeps the fascia from shortening and tightening too much during the night. When running, the large ground reaction forces place a heavy strain on the plantar fascia. Plantar fasciitis is also common in individuals with abnormal arches (too high or too low) and is typically caused by long runs, excessive downhill running, and lack of flexibility.

Achilles Tendinitis

This injury presents as a pain located in the Achilles tendon. When running, the triceps surae (gastrocnemius and soleus) is used heavily during plantar flexion of the toe-off phase. The triceps surae attaches to the posterior surface of the calcaneus via the Achilles tendon. Plantar flexion during running places a lot of strain on the tendon and can lead to Achilles tendinopathy. This condition is most commonly caused by too high an intensity or volume, lack of general flexibility, poor biomechanics, or heavy uphill running.

Iliotibial Band Syndrome

The tensor fascia latae originates on the iliac crest, runs downward on the lateral side of the leg, and ties into the iliotibial band (IT band), which inserts on the Gerdy's tubercle of the tibia. The IT band is a thick fascia of connective tissue that makes up most of the length from the iliac crest to the tibia. It is important that you can visualize the muscle and the IT band so that you can better understand IT band syndrome. The tensor fascia latae is used heavily in running as it is responsible for ensuring that the leg swings forward in a straight manner. The gluteus maximus places a large amount of strain on the IT band when running as it is used strongly during hip extension. To help avoid or eliminate IT band syndrome, work on hip and IT band flexibility.

Upper Body

In obstacle course racing and training, the upper body is used heavily when climbing and traversing overhead obstacles. As a result, upper body overuse injuries are common. Below I will discuss some of the more common upper body overuse injuries that you may encounter during training and racing.

Elbow Pain

Elbow pain can occur due to climbing, pull-ups, and overhead obstacles. The pain can either be centered around the outside of the elbow (commonly referred to as tennis elbow) or on the inside of the elbow (commonly referred to as golfer's elbow). Pain can stay local to the elbow or move up the forearm. These overuse injuries occur due to swelling and tendonitis from damage in the region of the elbow. Pain on the inside of the elbow is more common as it occurs due to gripping and hanging from objects. The best way to prevent tendonitis at the elbow is to strengthen the muscles of the forearm and to slowly work your way into obstacle course training.

Shoulder Pain

Obstacle course racing requires a large amount of overhead activity, which can result in shoulder pain. The muscles of the rotator cuff are designed to maintain static and dynamic stability of the humeral head within the glenoid fossa. Keep in mind that the muscles of the rotator cuff are small and easily fatigued. As the muscles and the ligaments of the shoulder become loose, the shoulder can subluxate, leading to tendinitis and muscular damage. In order to help prevent overuse injuries of the shoulder, it is important to work on muscular strength and muscular endurance to strengthen the muscles around the shoulder joint. Muscular imbalances also need to be addressed. Almost every obstacle requires a pulling motion, and therefore all muscles involved in pulling will be worked on a regular basis, whereas muscles involved in pushing are rarely worked. Make sure that you develop a well-balanced program. Also keep in mind that there are many different reasons for shoulder pain; it could be anything from impingement, to tendinitis, to a torn labrum, to a torn rotator cuff muscle. Any persistent pain should be evaluated by a doctor. This is especially true if you have pronounced weakness at the joint as well as pain.

Biceps Tendonitis

Bicep tendonitis can also occur in OCR athletes and presents as pain near the origin of the biceps brachii (long head: supraglenoid tubercle of the scapula, and short head: coracoid process of the scapula) or near the insertion of the biceps (radial tuberosity of the radius). A common location for bicep tendonitis is near the shoulder joint as the tendon of the long head passes through the bicipital groove of the humerus. This condition is often associated with shoulder pain. When the tendonitis is located near the elbow, it is more easily recognized as biceps tendonitis.

If caught early enough, most overuse injuries can be remedied before they become too severe. Rest, ice, and elevation can go a long way toward recovery. If approved by your doctor, over-the-counter anti-inflammatory medications can also help alleviate the pain. Do not ignore persistent pain as overuse injuries can progressively worsen over time. If pain worsens or does not go away, visit your doctor immediately.

EXERCISING IN THE HEAT

Training in the heat places a great amount of strain on the human body. Heat is generated as a byproduct of metabolism. As intensity increases, so too does metabolism, resulting in an increase in internal temperature. This internal heat generation during exercise, coupled with environmental heat, creates a very precarious situation.

The two forms of heat entering the body from the environment during training are radiation and conduction. Radiation is the primary method and is the transfer of heat through electromagnetic waves. The sun provides radiant heat and is the most common form of heat. Radiation from the sun can either be direct or reflected off objects, such as asphalt. During the summer, thermal ground heat will radiate upward and can be transferred to the body during training. Conduction is not experienced to a large degree during training as it requires direct molecular contact in order for heat to transfer. The most common form of conduction during training is when the foot makes contact with the hot ground.

In order to prevent a heat-related illness, it is important to dissipate heat effectively from the body. In order for the body to dispel heat through radiation, the body temperature must be higher than the environmental temperature, not always an option. Conduction is not an effective method for heat dissipation during exercise either. Therefore, the two main sources for heat dissipation during exercise are convection and evaporation. Convection is the transfer of heat through a fluid medium. As the air travels across the body, the boundary layer of air next to the skin is continuously replaced with cooler air. The faster the boundary layer is replaced, the faster the body can dissipate heat. This is how fans work to help keep the body cool during exercise.

Evaporation of sweat on the skin transfers heat to the environment and is the primary method of heat dissipation during exercise. In order for the cooling process to occur, the sweat must evaporate on the skin. Relative humidity (the ratio of water contained in the air compared to the amount the air could contain) affects the ability of the human body to cool through the use of evaporation. If the relative humidity is 60 percent, then 40 percent of the air can accept the water. If the relative humidity is 90 percent, then only 10 percent of the air can absorb water, leaving little room for evaporation to occur and negatively impacting evaporative cooling during exercise. Windy days are beneficial as air moving across the skin will continually replace the boundary layer with less-saturated air to aid in cooling.

During exercise, heat is generated by the working muscles, increasing both muscle temperature and core temperature. In order for cooling to occur, the heat must be transferred from the muscles and core to the skin so that it may be dissipated into the surrounding environment. Blood makes an excellent transporter of heat as roughly 50 to 55 percent of blood consists of water. Autoregulation of blood flow allows for the redirection of blood flow to the skin in order to dissipate heat through evaporation, convection, and radiation. The cooled blood will then recirculate through the body to pick up more heat, and the process repeats. Keep in mind that as heat increases, a greater amount of blood flow will be redirected to the skin. This lowers the volume of blood flow to the working muscles and reduces performance.

As you can see, blood is vital in the process of heat dissipation. As blood is made up of predominantly water, hydration status strongly impacts the body's ability to cool. When you become dehydrated, your ability to cool the body is strongly impacted. To make a long story short, sweat is filtered plasma, and as you sweat plasma volume decreases. The decrease in plasma volume results in dehydration and impaired cooling. As your ability to dissipate heat becomes compromised, the core temperature begins to steadily rise, resulting in the development of a heat-related illness. Water loss equivalent to 2 to 3 percent of body mass will negatively impact performance, whereas a loss equivalent to 5 percent or greater will negatively impact health. These numbers assume that you began the session fully hydrated.

Heat-Related Illnesses

Heat-related illness occurs when the body's ability to dissipate heat has been compromised due to high internal and external temperatures and dehydration. Heat-related illnesses are of serious concern and can result in death if untreated. As an obstacle course racer, there are many discomforts or pains that you can push through (I do not advise this course of action). However, a heat-related illness is not one of them. The primary heat-related illnesses are heat cramps, heat exhaustion, and heat stroke.

Heat Cramps

Heat cramps present as very strong and painful muscle contractions, which occur due to dehydration and sodium loss. The best way to counter heat cramps is to stop exercising, get to a cool environment, rehydrate, and ingest electrolytes.

Heat Exhaustion

As your ability to dissipate heat continues to diminish, the thermoregulatory system is unable to effectively dissipate heat. The primary symptoms of heat exhaustion are as follows:

- headache
- dizziness
- nausea
- feeling of weakness
- tingling sensation in the skin
- chills
- pale, moist skin
- rapid, weak pulse

Heat Stroke

As you progress beyond heat exhaustion, your ability to dissipate heat is further impacted, resulting in heat stroke. Of the three heat-related illnesses, heat stroke is the worst as it can cause serious health issues, including death. Some of the heat stroke symptoms are the same as those found in heat exhaustion. There are a few key symptoms that differ, however, the most important of which is the development of a core temperature of 104°F or higher. The other differing symptoms are cessation of sweating and hot, red, dry skin; these are signs that you have moved from heat exhaustion to heat stroke. The full list of the symptoms of heat stroke are:

- core temperature greater than or equal to 104°F
- hot, red, dry skin
- cessation of sweating
- rapid, strong pulse
- headache
- dizziness
- nausea
- feeling of weakness
- tingling sensation in the skin
- confusion
- chills

At the first sign of a heat-related illness, you should stop exercising immediately, cool the body down as quickly as possible, and drink plenty of fluids. As heat-related injuries can escalate in severity in a very quick progression, it is important to cease activity immediately upon the first signs. Once core temperature starts to increase beyond the body's ability to control it, it will continue to rise as long as you exercise and generate metabolic heat in a hot environment.

Once you have ceased activity and have moved into a cooler environment, continue working to bring the core temperature down. There are methods you can use to lower core temperature to normal levels, such as taking a cool shower or bath, applying cold towels, or using ice packs. As dehydration is a key component of heat-related illnesses, it is also very important to ingest fluids. Rehydration can become problematic when you are nauseous and cannot keep fluids down. If this is the case, a trip to the doctor and an IV will most likely be required. If you suspect that you have heat stroke, seek medical attention immediately.

Prevention

Here are a few basic prevention strategies that will help you avoid heat-related illnesses. When training outside, avoid the hottest part of the day and instead train early before the temperatures get too high. If training indoors, try to keep the temperature as cool as possible and use fans.

Choose appropriate clothing when training in the heat. Clothing should be breathable so that sweat is able to evaporate on the skin in order to cool the body. When training outside, do not wear dark colors as they will absorb radiation from the sun to a much greater extent than lighter colors.

As stated previously, proper hydration is important for dissipating heat and maintaining a functioning core temperature. Unfortunately, most athletes are chronically dehydrated during the summertime due to long hours training and inadequate hydration strategies. Keep track of water loss and water ingestion in order to help maintain proper hydration levels. Check your weight before and after training to determine water loss, and replace each pound lost with approximately 24 ounces of fluid.

Acclimatization is the strongest step that you can take to help prevent a heat-related illness. It will take approximately two weeks of training in the heat for significant physiological changes to occur during the acclimatization process. As the body adapts to the heat, more blood will be directed to the skin for cooling and there will be a more efficient distribution of blood throughout the body. There will be significant alterations to sweating; you will begin to sweat more, sweat will start at a lower core temperature, and sweat will be better distributed across the body to optimize cooling. Sodium concentrations within sweat will decrease in order to help offset electrolyte imbalances that occur during heavy sodium loss. Glycogen usage significantly increases when exercising in the heat. After acclimation, glycogen usage will not be as high as prior to acclimation. This will spare glycogen stores, which are limited and can negatively impact performance when diminished.

In order to appropriately acclimate to training in the heat, you should start slowly and train during cooler parts of the day. Do not attempt to acclimate by training during the hottest part of the day or by conducting high-volume or high-intensity bouts in the heat. Instead, start increasing volume and intensity after the two-week acclimation period.

INDEX

ABOUT THE AUTHOR

Will Peveler is a noted physiologist with a teaching and research focus on the physiological and biomechanical factors that influence sport performance and is professor of exercise science at Liberty University. Dr. Peveler has a strong background in endurance sports and experience in obstacle course racing. He was a diver on active duty with the U.S. Navy and Army and a drill sergeant in the reserves. He is the author of the Train Like a Pro book series, *The Complete Book of Road Cycling*, and *Racing and Triathlon Training Fundamentals*.

www.ingramcontent.com/pod-product-compliance
Lightning Source LLC
Chambersburg PA
CBHW030310100426
42812CB00002B/650